W9-ABM-982

SASKATOON PUBLIC LIBRARY
36001404913622
CBD : self-care secrets to hemp-derived

RITUAL WELLNESS

CBD

Self-Care Secrets to Hemp-Derived Wellness

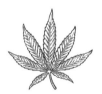

Blair Lauren Brown
Founder of Verté Essentials

Foreword by Chelsea Leyland

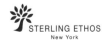

STERLING ETHOS
New York

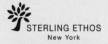

STERLING ETHOS
New York

An Imprint of Sterling Publishing Co., Inc.
1166 Avenue of the Americas
New York, NY 10036

STERLING ETHOS and the distinctive Sterling logo are registered
trademarks of Sterling Publishing Co.

Interior text © 2020 Blair Lauren Brown
Cover © 2020 Sterling Publishing Co., Inc.

All rights reserved. No part of this publication may be reproduced, stored in a retrieval system,
or transmitted in any form or by any means (including electronic, mechanical, photocopying,
recording, or otherwise) without prior written permission from the publisher.

This publication is intended for informational purposes only, and the publisher does not claim that
this publication shall provide or guarantee any benefits, healing, cure, or any results in any respect.
This publication includes alternative therapies that have not been scientifically tested and is not
intended to provide or replace conventional medical advice, treatment, or diagnosis or be a substitute
to consulting with licensed health-care providers. The publisher shall not be liable or responsible in
any respect for any use or application of any content contained in this publication or any adverse
effects, consequence, loss, or damage of any type resulting or arising from, directly or indirectly,
such use or application. Any trademarks are the property of their respective owners, are used
for editorial purposes only, and the publisher makes no claim of ownership and shall acquire
no right, title or interest in such trademarks by virtue of this publication.

ISBN 978-1-4549-3463-9

Distributed in Canada by Sterling Publishing Co., Inc.
c/o Canadian Manda Group, 664 Annette Street
Toronto, Ontario M6S 2C8, Canada
Distributed in the United Kingdom by GMC Distribution Services
Castle Place, 166 High Street, Lewes, East Sussex BN7 1XU, England
Distributed in Australia by NewSouth Books
University of New South Wales, Sydney, NSW 2052, Australia

For information about custom editions, special sales, and premium and corporate
purchases, please contact Sterling Special Sales at 800-805-5489 or
specialsales@sterlingpublishing.com.

Manufactured in Canada

2 4 6 8 10 9 7 5 3 1

sterlingpublishing.com

Cover design by David Ter-Avanesyan
Cover photography © Aubrey Lu Nova
Interior design by Ashley Prine, Tandem Books

For picture credits, see page 151

CONTENTS

FOREWORD

I have been battling juvenile myoclonic epilepsy since my early teens. One evening, during a casual conversation with some friends, a cannabis advocate that I'd known for some time mentioned that CBD provided some relief for epilepsy patients.

I started taking medication for epilepsy when I was about fifteen years old. The side effects were numerous, including insomnia, which ironically happens to be a trigger for epilepsy. The only thing worse than the side effects was the anxiety of living with epilepsy and not knowing when the next seizure would occur. My neurologist prescribed medication and supported its use. When I tried to address its side effects, there were no alternatives presented. I struggled a lot with them. This struggle led to depression and overwhelm, and at times even made me feel suicidal.

So, I tried a few drops of a CBD tincture. The effects were instantaneous, which is something that still seems to surprise me when I say it out loud. I even forgot to take my epilepsy medicine that evening, which I would never forget to do. Nothing previously ever needed to remind me to take my pills, as my brain would do that for me. Forgetting them that night was a profound indication that I was onto something and that there was something deeper to explore here.

Discovering CBD was like being plugged into a power source, as though I had been Humpty Dumpty for all these years, and this new medicine was now putting all my little pieces back together again. I began to experience feelings of wholeness and balance.

This was the beginning of a very colorful and textured experience with CBD. CBD has not only given me back my life but also allowed me to wean myself off all my pharmaceuticals. I felt like I owed my life to this plant. I had never had a calling as intense as wanting to help other patients gain access to it, or at least learn and have the option to try this medicine.

CBD has the potential to help many people. It is not just about patients like me, who use it for epilepsy. While there may not be masses of scientific evidence on its use for many health conditions, there is anecdotal evidence. There is an abundance of people who are using CBD for many different ailments. The medical applications are already beyond what we first perceived.

Before I met Blair, through a mutual friend in the cannabis industry, I had tried a product from her apothecary line, Verté Essentials. I saw an intelligence rooted in both science and nature behind the product. For a market largely unregulated, quality is important. That intelligence is applied to all Blair's endeavors, including this book.

This impressive and beautiful guide brings such a feminine and tender tone to a very wide-reaching exploration into the landscape of cannabis. I love the moments when Blair invites the audience in by setting the scene and illustrating an experience. She presents CBD as something that you can imagine yourself using and she offers people incredibly empowering information. I love all the recipes she's included—they bring a certain earthy magic to the whole experience of exploring this plant, allowing the reader to learn that people and plants do, after all, speak the same "phyto-language." This book is delicately well-balanced with a soft, nurturing essence that is just what is needed right now.

Chelsea Leyland is a British DJ and medical cannabis/epilepsy activist based in Brooklyn, New York. In 2016, Chelsea made the brave and life-changing decision to wean herself off her strong pharmaceutical anti-seizure medications and treat her epilepsy solely with medical cannabis. She has used her experiences and her platform to become a leading advocate for the destigmatization of both epilepsy and medical cannabis. Through her advocacy work, she has spoken on multiple medical cannabis panels, given talks, and has appeared on teaching podcasts. Chelsea is now producing Separating the Strains, *a documentary that explores the medical cannabis landscape in both the UK and the US, as well as her fight to gain access to this treatment for her older sister, Tamsin.*

INTRODUCTION

Cannabidiol, also known as CBD, is cannabis's (currently) most sought after molecule because of the value it has within and beyond its physical and psychological healing properties. In this book, you'll find out what it is, what it does, and how to use it.

I come to this space of expert knowledge with sincere reverence, even with almost twenty years of experience working with cannabis under my belt. My journey began with my immediate family. My grandfather, a Stanford MD and the sixth generation of doctors in my family, had prescribed my mother cannabis to aid in her cancer recovery. My own entrée into the world of cannabis was slow and calculated. While I had been around cannabis for years because of my mother's cancer recovery, I didn't touch it in a professional capacity because I was uncertain about how it might affect my world.

I felt that cannabis was too taboo, and that my career ambitions could be compromised by judgmental peers and legal uncertainty. Instead, I watched from the sidelines and took in what the California community and my brother Jay, an organic medicinal cannabis grower and consultant, was doing after the 1996 passage of Proposition 215, which legalized medical cannabis in the state. I only helped in ways where I could keep cannabis at arm's length. In 2016, when the majority of states in the US legalized medical cannabis, I decided it was time. I founded, and own, one of the first wellness companies focused on CBD, Verté Essentials.

Originally, the plan was to develop products that use the whole cannabis plant, which has a wide range of compounds, including THC. But, after meticulous research, I discovered that my team and I could expand our reach and create the products we wanted with CBD and other complementary plant botanicals. After early testing with friends and family and then a wider network of people, I found that these products achieved desirable benefits, from deeper sleep to reduced inflammation, from anxiety relief to a diminishment of pain.

I also wanted to create something that honors the past and embraces our future. There is no question that cannabis deserves a spotlight today, but it is also important to honor its history. That is why this book will not just talk about CBD but also cannabis as a whole—to help you understand the context behind this single compound and why it's suddenly everywhere. It will help you understand the conversation at large around cannabis. It gives you the information you need to make the best choices not only for your personal consumption but also for supporting the cannabis community and building a sustainable market that operates with integrity and supports safe cannabis medicines and remedies, environmentally considerate agricultural practices, ethical product development, social equity programs, and much, much more.

It is important to note that cannabis and CBD haven't yet been the subjects of extensive scientific data and field studies (most of which is still restricted to lab and animal testing in the US) because of its lengthy prohibition, which has gone on for as long as eighty years in some countries. That leaves us with a small handful of studies, historical accounts of CBD's efficacy, and the experiences of present-day CBD users. I will share the formal research to give you a backbone of scientific knowledge, but I will also review the history of cannabis's medicinal uses. Members of the cannabis community, including leading experts in CBD research, cannabis advocates, and other health and wellness specialists, have contributed to this book, sharing everything from home remedies to personal rituals for connecting with the plant and their bodies.

This guide offers an opportunity to uncover the diversity of applications presented by the ancient and ever-evolving experience of CBD. You'll quickly learn how CBD is one of many tools that can be used in any wellness practice.

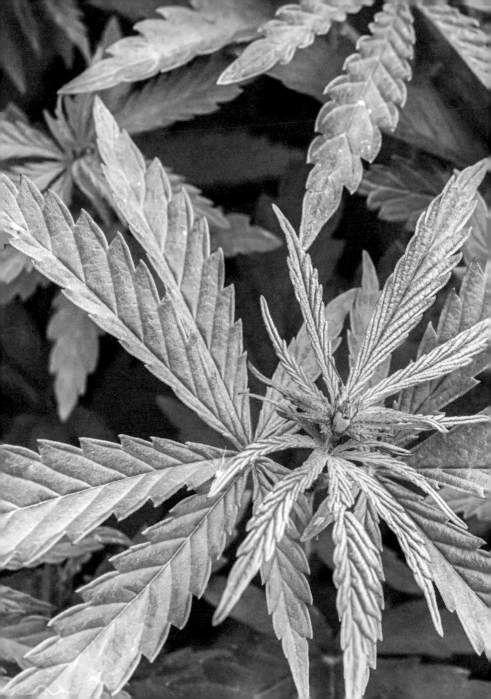

CHAPTER ONE

The Story of Cannabis

The story of cannabis is complex. Though it is a plant like any other, grown and nurtured by the sun and soil, it has been used in medicinal and industrial applications. In less than a hundred years' time, it has been criminalized and decriminalized. Here, I will provide a brief window into the six-thousand-year history of cannabis, illustrate how cannabis has been stigmatized, and address the recent events surrounding the decriminalization of cannabis and the rise of CBD.

THE CANNABIS PLANT

While you might just simply want to understand CBD and its applications, it is important to get the full picture of cannabis. Understanding the distinctions between different types of cannabis will help you understand the history of the plant, and, in turn, make informed decisions about any CBD product you engage with.

You may already be privy to the differences between the two most-talked-about varieties, cannabis and hemp. They both come from the same plant species, *Cannabis sativa*, but they vary slightly in their chemical makeup. Thus, they have been cultivated for different purposes, cannabis for its psychoactive properties and hemp primarily for industrial use.

Cannabis is a bushy plant that has been primarily cultivated for its flowers, which is where you find the concentration of THC (delta-9-tetrahydrocannabinol), among other compounds. Cannabis has been used for the treatment of epilepsy, glaucoma, multiple sclerosis, cancer, the effects of strokes, and post-traumatic stress disorder (PTSD), to name just a few.

Hemp, on the other hand, has historically been grown for its fiber, and it is cultivated in tall, densely packed fields where plants appear in a crop-like bamboo formation. Hemp is used to make more

CANNABIS OR MARIJUANA?

Where I use the term *cannabis*, some will use the term *marijuana*. Moving forward, I will only refer to the plant as cannabis. Marijuana (also spelled "marihuana") is the Spanish term for cannabis, though there are different theories on where the word originated. It came onto the scene to describe smokable cannabis in the 1930s. It was then used to associate cannabis with negative stereotypes of Mexican immigrants in the US. I will go into detail about that later, on page 10. I see marijuana as a term of marginalization that perpetuates a system I am not interested in supporting. I hope you, too, will join me and eliminate it from your vocabulary.

than 25,000 products, including food, clothing, building materials, cars, biodegradable plastic, and body products, and it has medicinal applications as well.

The most notable difference between cannabis and hemp is that hemp presents with less THC and a larger concentration of CBD, while cannabis presents a larger quantity of THC and much smaller quantities of CBD. THC and CBD are cannabinoids, the active molecules found in cannabis, each playing different roles individually and synergistically. THC creates a psychoactive response—it's what gets you high and interacts with neurotransmitters—whereas CBD is a powerful anti-inflammatory agent that has anti-anxiety properties and helps with wound healing. There are potentially hundreds of cannabinoids in cannabis, though we are familiar only with around a hundred of them.

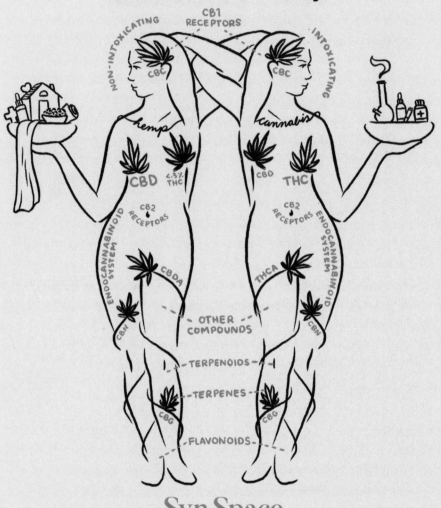

KEY COMPOUNDS IN CANNABIS

This list presents an overview of the key compounds referenced in the diagram. You'll find more information about the endocannabinoid system and CB1 and CB2 receptors in chapter 2.

CBD: cannabidiol; nonpsychoactive; may relieve inflammation, anxiety, and pain

THC: tetrahydrocannabinol; psychoactive; has intoxicating effects, may relieve chronic pain, depression, eating disorders, and many other conditions

CBN: cannabinol; mildly psychoactive; may relieve inflammation and may be an antibiotic

CBG: cannabigerol; nonpsychoactive; may relieve inflammation, pain, and nausea

CBC: cannabichromene; nonpsychoactive; supports function of other cannabinoids, potential cancer fighter

CBDA: cannabidiolic acid; live or raw, unheated CBD; supports function of other cannabinoids, potentially relieves inflammation

THCA: tetrahydrocannabinolic acid; live or raw, unheated THC; supports function of other cannabinoids, potentially has neuroprotective properties

Terpenes and terpenoids: aromatic compounds; potentially enhance physical and mental states as well as the effect of other cannabinoids

Flavonoids: natural plant chemicals that color the plant; potentially have antioxidant properties

The diagram on page 4 summarizes the similarities and differences of CBD-dominant and THC-dominant cannabis. The potential benefits of each active molecule are too numerous to mention, so we have highlighted a few of the most talked about. I go into further detail in chapter 2 about what these benefits are and how they function.

Current regulations in the US distinguish hemp from cannabis by its THC content. Cannabis with less than 0.3 percent of THC can be classified under the 2018 Farm Bill as hemp and sold on a national marketplace, with a few exceptions depending on individual state regulations. You can find other types of CBD-rich cannabis but with varying amounts of THC in regulated markets for medical cannabis, again, depending on the state. Canada has fully legalized cannabis under the Cannabis Act; however, there are variations on the laws from province to province. CBD in Canada is regulated and sold only by licensed manufacturers in the country. Most international laws legally recognize CBD only if it is derived from hemp plants. The EU employs this distinction almost universally with the exception of a few countries. It also requires that CBD products contain less than 0.2 percent THC. In Japan, CBD extracts with 0 percent THC are legal. In China, CBD is legal for use in cosmetics, but they have not ruled on other types of CBD consumption. If I were to go on country by country, we would be here forever, so if you are traveling or a resident of one of these countries, I would suggest you look up the local laws from a trusted source.

A BRIEF HISTORY OF CANNABIS USE

Cannabis has appeared in a variety of geographical locations and cultures across time. Texts on Ayurveda, India's traditional practice of medicine, record cannabis use as far back as 2000 BCE. Ayurveda was founded on the belief that the body is a fully integrated system requiring balance, not just from herbs and medicine but also from diet, breath, mind, and spirit. Cannabis use was accepted as a religious practice, which facilitated the exploration of its medical benefits. Cannabis was documented as a treatment for ailments including aches and pains, digestion issues, and anxiety. The Vedas, for example, described cannabis as a "joy-giver."

In the Chinese historical record, cannabis shows up time and again in the *Shen-nung pen-ts'ao ching*, a text on traditional Chinese medicine text referenced as far back as 4000 BCE. Recorded use can be found in other parts of the world with nomadic Indo-European people using cannabis in baths, and in the Egyptian text "Ebers Papyrus" from 1550 BCE, which mentions using cannabis to treat inflammation. Populations across the African continent and the ancient Roman elite alike have used cannabis in birthing rituals to relieve labor pains.

Documented medical use of cannabis continues across continents into the eighteenth century as doctors began to address ailments on a chemical basis and focus on managing symptoms. These depictions of cannabis use range from analgesic effects described by the Chinese physician Hua To in 207 CE, to *The Canon of Medicine* by the Persian medical writer Avicenna in 1025, to the work of the nineteenth-century Irish physician William Brooke O'Shaughnessy, who introduced cannabis's therapeutic uses to Western medicine. Medicinal use of cannabis began appearing in Western culture in the early 1900s when pharmaceutical companies such as Bristol-Myers Squibb and Eli Lilly started offering medicines that contained cannabis or cannabis extracts.

Hemp's industrial applications also have a long history. There are more than 22,000 different uses for hemp seeds, flowers, and stalks. Paper is one of the oldest forms of industrial hemp fiber use on record. In

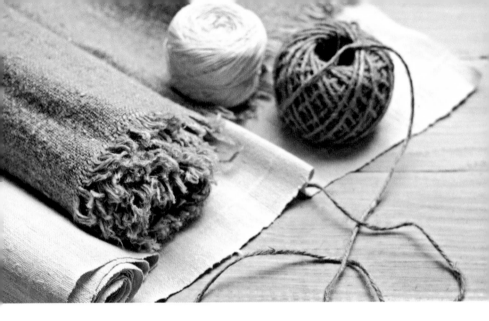

fact, many ancient texts were largely written on hemp paper. Hemp has also been used to produce fibrous materials such as rope and clothing. Hemp cloth dating as far back as 8000 BCE has been discovered in what was once ancient Mesopotamia, and Chinese texts from 500 CE teach hemp cultivation for the purposes of making cloth.

Later accounts across Europe and the Americas describe hemp as one of the, if not *the*, most important materials for the production of canvas rope and other fiber products. The word *canvas* is thought to be derived from the word *cannabis*. In 1535, King Henry VIII even penalized landowners for not growing at least a quarter acre of hemp. These examples are not the only representations of hemp's importance, but they paint a picture of how the plant's story spans continents and how unanimously hemp was appreciated.

In the 1930s, hemp was still used in many products. Imagine that you are in that decade. One morning you read the paper and see an advertisement for a new feature at the local movie theater. You head to the theater and buy some popcorn, which you now have in hand as you wait for the picture to start. Ropes are draped in front of the screen to keep children from touching the projections. The lights go black as you hear the sounds of the projector start to roll. Before the film has even begun, there have likely been at least three examples of cannabis use. The newspaper could have been made from hemp paper. Hemp fibers could have been used to stitch your trousers, as well as to make the rope across the stage. You might have even taken a cannabis tincture designed to soothe indigestion after eating all the popcorn.

The Prohibition of Cannabis

Though many people used cannabis-derived products every single day, the US imposed a tax on hemp cultivation in 1937 in the Marihuana Tax Act. This tax was imposed on anyone who sold or cultivated the cannabis plant, making it increasingly cost-prohibitive to be involved in the business. What changed government policy and, eventually, people's minds about cannabis?

In 1930, President Herbert Hoover appointed Harry J. Anslinger as the first director of the recently created Federal Bureau of Narcotics (now the Drug Enforcement Agency, or DEA). Formed in 1930 under the Department of the Treasury, the Federal Bureau of Narcotics was put in place to fight opium and heroin trafficking. Holding office for thirty years, Anslinger was one of the predominant figures in the stigmatization of cannabis. Under the guise of controlling addiction, he helped create an anti-cannabis campaign that also promoted racist and anti-immigrant views and shaped the language used to discuss cannabis.

Enter the term *marijuana*—the Latino-Spanish word for cannabis. Prior to the 1900s, *cannabis* was used to refer to the plant in news reports and medical journals, and smoking cannabis recreationally was a pastime reserved for the mainly white, social elite during parties and in other celebratory settings. The Mexican Revolution, which began in 1910, sent a wave of immigrants across the US–Mexico border, and they introduced the word *marijuana* to Americans. Anti-cannabis politicians as well as major media outlets began to popularize the usage of *marijuana* and negatively associate the drug with Mexican immigrants. Ultimately, by not using the word *cannabis* to refer to the plant, anti-cannabis factions could create a stigma around the plant that didn't exist before.

Many newspapers published articles using the newly discovered word *marijuana*, describing how cannabis use led to violence and addiction, and portraying it as a drug of choice for many marginalized groups, from Mexican immigrants to African Americans to sex workers. The *New York Times* ran a headline in February 1925 that read "Kills Six in a Hospital. Mexican Crazed by Marihuana, Runs Amuck with Butcher Knife." The *Seattle Daily* ran a sensational headline from March 16, 1913: "Evil Mexican Plants That Drive You Insane." The article goes on to explain, "The revolution in Mexico has brought with it not only the ravages of war, but also the degradation of the social conditions of soldiers and prisoners. One of the latest forms of dissipation on the ranks of federals and rebels alike is the habit of smoking marihuana, a deadly native plant to Mexico. According to reports many of the Mexican prisoners in the Belem prison in the City of Mexico are losing their minds as a result of smoking this weed." In 1936, the propaganda film *Reefer Madness* was released. It depicted fictionalized caricatures of drug dealers luring children to the dark side of "reefer" smoking culture, perpetuating every stereotype of cannabis portrayed in the press. Originally produced and paid for by a church group called Tell Your Children, it soon stigmatized cannabis use and became a weapon in

Anslinger's campaign to create more-uniform drug enforcement policies across the United States.

As the media spread stereotypes and tabloid-style headlines about the "marijuana menace," policymakers and appointed officials shared similar racist sentiments that supported the sensationalized media reports. Anslinger proclaimed before Congress while presenting the Marihuana Tax Act of 1937, "Marijuana is the most violence-causing drug in the history of mankind. . . . Most marijuana smokers are Negroes, Hispanics, Filipinos, and entertainers. Their satanic music, jazz and swing, result from marijuana usage." He later wrote, "Reefer makes darkies think they're as good as white men. . . . The primary reason to outlaw marijuana is its effect on the degenerate races."

The Marihuana Tax Act of 1937 laid the groundwork for the prohibition of cannabis in the US on a federal level by effectively halting its cultivation, even as a 1938 issue of *Popular Mechanics* hailed hemp as the "new billion-dollar crop" due to the introduction of new production and harvesting equipment. Just as the plant was starting to be recognized for its great value to the nation, it was also being cut down because of its unsavory reputation.

It is possible that the rise of hemp may have posed a threat to chemical and agricultural industries, so some corporations may have had interests in controlling or stifling hemp production. For example, DuPont, the largest chemical manufacturer in the US, had patented synthetic fiber production in 1938, creating an alternative to hemp textiles, which had made up 80 percent of all apparel until the 1920s. Hearst, the largest publishing company in the US at the time, maintained significant holdings in cotton and lumber, hemp's competitors in paper production.

The public perception of cannabis had effectively been altered and it was now seen as a dangerous, addictive drug. This influenced policies and laws on the state, federal, and even international level. By the 1930s, many states in the US had banned cannabis, some doing so by classifying cannabis alongside already regulated narcotics. Beginning in 1961, a total of 155 countries signed the first international treaty prohibiting the production and supply of cannabis along with other hard drugs, like cocaine and heroin, with some exceptions for cannabis used for medicinal purposes. In 1970, under US President Richard Nixon, Congress passed the Controlled Substances Act, creating a standardized classification system that categorized drugs based on their potential for abuse. These classifications are referred to as "schedules" with Schedule I being the most addictive and dangerous and Schedule V being the least. Cannabis was labeled a Schedule I drug, along with cocaine, heroin, and morphine. After the passage of the Controlled Substances Act, it officially no longer recognized industrial hemp and medicinal "marijuana" as two separate varieties of the cannabis plant.

The next year, President Richard Nixon began his all-out "war on drugs." Despite unanimous recommendations by a drug enforcement commission in 1972, Nixon refused to decriminalize possession of cannabis for personal use. With the creation of the Drug Enforcement Administration (DEA) in 1973, the US government had a streamlined process for generating and enforcing policies related to drug laws, and funding for drug-fighting campaigns increased. Thousands were imprisoned for nonviolent drug offenses, and many drug enforcement efforts disproportionately affected people of color in the following decades.

In the 1980s, President Ronald Regan continued to take a harsh stance on drug enforcement. With the implementation of new mandatory minimum sentencing laws for the use and possession of several drugs, including cannabis, incarceration rates soared further. Meanwhile, First Lady Nancy Reagan began her "Just Say No" campaign to teach children about the dangers of drugs. In 1984, despite the lack of substantial or clinical evidence, cannabis was presented as a "gateway" drug that led to the eventual abuse of narcotics.

The drug enforcement policies of the 1970s and beyond have been seen as a response to the anti-establishment sentiments and rising political dissent in the 1960s. John Ehrlichman, a domestic policy chief during the Nixon administration, later described the war on drugs as a campaign motivated by these factors. He said, "You want to know what this was really all about? The Nixon campaign in 1968, and the Nixon White House after that, had two enemies: the antiwar left and black people. . . . We knew we couldn't make it illegal to be either against the war or black, but by getting the public to associate the hippies with marijuana and blacks with heroin, and then criminalizing both heavily, we could disrupt those communities. We could arrest their leaders, raid their homes, break up their meetings, and vilify them night after night on the evening news. Did we know we were lying about the drugs? Of course we did." The policies that came out of the war on drugs left a destructive legacy, harming many communities, hampering research on medical cannabis, and severely restricting access to a plant that has been used for centuries.

Legalization of Medical Cannabis

Despite having been stigmatized legally and in the popular imagination, researchers were studying cannabis in the US and around the world. In 1963–1964, Raphael Mechoulam, an organic chemist and professor of medicinal chemistry at the Hebrew University of Jerusalem who became known as the "father of cannabis," isolated THC. In 1988, Allyn Howlett and William Devane, researchers working with government funding in the US, uncovered the existence of cannabinoid receptors in the brains of rats. Working in Mechoulam's lab in 1992, Lumír Hanuš and William Devane isolated the first known endocannabinoid in the human brain. They named it *anandamide*, confirming that the human brain produces cannabinoids on its own, which then bind with cannabinoid receptors throughout the brain and body. Their subsequent research uncovered more cannabinoids. Uncovering the cannabinoids and the receptors led to the discovery of the endocannabinoid system (ECS). The researchers learned that the ECS helps maintain homeostasis (balance) in the body.

It wasn't until the 1980s AIDS epidemic that the US began to consider legalizing medical cannabis. In a scenario where no cure presented itself, cannabis seemed to provide relief from some of the symptoms of HIV including pain, nausea, and lack of appetite, and so law enforcement turned the other cheek for a while. Dennis Peron, a Vietnam War veteran, was moved to help his partner who was suffering from the disease. He created the first medical cannabis dispensary, called the San Francisco Buyers Club. Peron went on to cowrite Proposition 215 with several other activists and professionals. Passed in 1996, Proposition 215 was the first bill to legalize cannabis for medical use and made California the first state to do so.

With the passage of Prop 215, legalization efforts and the decriminalization of cannabis picked up steam in the US and other countries, including Uruguay and Portugal among others. There was also renewed interest from both the public and scientific community in cannabis's medical applications. In the US, one of the most profound stories that helped increase access to cannabis and shone a spotlight on CBD is that of Charlotte Figi. At age 5, Charlotte Figi suffered from over three hundred seizures a day, affecting her ability to walk, talk, and develop as a normal child. Despite years of trying every possible medical treatment, nothing helped Charlotte or diminished her seizure count. In

"I use cannabis as a conduit for larger discussions. The multi-faceted nature of the plant touches on many subjects from health and environmental impact to public policy. We are at a pivotal moment in history. Through breaking the chains of prohibition—and recognizing the harm inflicted by the war on drugs—we have a once-in-a-generation opportunity to flip many social paradigms, crafting a future narrative for the cannabis industry that is equitable, fair, and regenerative."

—Danniel Swatosh,
  cofounder of Humble Bloom

2000, Colorado established a medical cannabis registry program allowing limited access to cannabis for very specific conditions including cancer, HIV/AIDS, muscle spasms, seizures, severe pain, and nausea. Conventional medical wisdom presented cannabis as unsafe for children, but after considerable challenges, Charlotte's parents found doctors in Colorado who prescribed medical cannabis for their daughter. Working with a dispensary in Denver, the Figis found a strain of cannabis, high in CBD and low in THC, that nearly eliminated Charlotte's seizures. By six years old, she was riding a bike and learning to talk. The strain of cannabis used to help Charlotte was named Charlotte's Web by the Stanley Brothers, the men who had created it. This story of a parent's last hope, combined with the media spotlight that it received and the great success of the treatment, began to open conversations about destigmatizing cannabis and shined a spotlight on CBD's therapeutic potential.

CANNABIS IN THE PRESENT DAY

As of this writing, thirty-three states have legalized cannabis for just medical use, and eleven for the adult-use market. US patent 6630507B1 recognizes cannabinoids as antioxidants and neurological protectants. In June 2018, the Food and Drug Administration (FDA) approved Epidiolex, the first drug containing CBD for the treatment of severe cases of epilepsy. Six months later, the passage of the Farm Bill legalized hemp cannabis, removing its Schedule I designation and acknowledging it as an agricultural commodity. These developments with hemp have helped cannabis take its initial steps toward becoming destigmatized and have opened the door to making cannabis products, especially CBD products, more accessible. Internationally, we are starting to see a similar move toward legalization and the destigmatizing of cannabis. Since the start of the 2000s, there are twenty-six countries where cannabis possession is not a punishable offense, and Argentina even offers medical cannabis to patients for free.

The criminalization of cannabis took place over many years at the expense of many communities. The reintegration of cannabis into our daily lives will require careful navigation. Legalization of cannabis presents a host of questions. What does decriminalization mean for every industry it touches, for every person it impacts, and for international relations? What does creating access to cannabis look like from the point of view of the farmer, the government official, or someone who was incarcerated for a cannabis-related offense? What does it mean to change our minds about cannabis after the Marihuana Tax Act or the war on drugs? What would happen if farmers used industrial agricultural practices to grow cannabis? How do farmers, business owners, and consumers handle new regulations? How does the cannabis industry develop with consideration for its social, environmental, and political impacts?

For now, we have CBD. Though we may not be able to answer all these questions or have access to the whole plant and all its healing properties today, CBD allows us to begin exploring cannabis and participating in a larger conversation about cannabis.

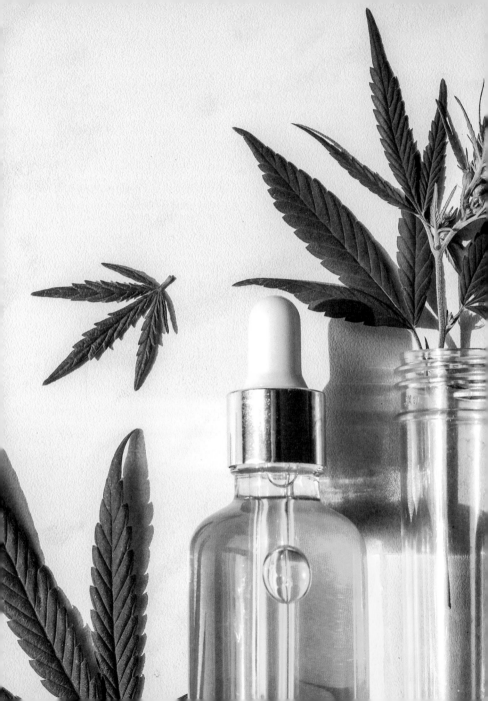

· CHAPTER TWO ·

CBD and
the Body

Throughout history, cannabis has been used to treat various conditions, especially before the advent of modern science and Western medicine. It is still used in places where people don't have access to Western medicine—and increasingly in places where they do. Evidence of the plant's beneficial attributes have traditionally come down from first-hand experiences, but today we know more about the science behind cannabis and how it affects our bodies.

PHYTONUTRIENTS

While we are focusing on the cannabidiol, or CBD, molecule and its benefits, it is important not to overlook the properties and benefits of the whole cannabis plant, as you won't often see the CBD molecule by itself. It is possible to purchase the isolate to use alone, but most products combine isolated CBD with other complementary plant ingredients. Certain combinations of molecules from the cannabis plant and complementary ingredients work together to enhance the effect of the CBD. If you refer back to the SVN Space diagram in chapter 1 (page 4), you can see that key compounds—flavonoids and terpenes, among others—are present in all types of cannabis. These compounds are also present in roses, lemon trees, strawberries, and every other plant under the sun.

Plants produce a variety of these key compounds to protect themselves from environmental harm. These are called *phytonutrients* (*phyto* is Latin for "plant"). Through time, scientists have found that these phytonutrients have the same protective powers for humans: They're antioxidizing, or cell protecting; anti-inflammatory; analgesic, or pain-relieving; relaxing; and much more. Take the delicate but sturdy damask rose, for instance. Its compounds have been found to help protect human cells from cancer, or if cancer is already present, to keep it from spreading. Let's take a closer look at some of these compounds.

Flavonoids

Flavonoids are part of a class of phytonutrients called *polyphenols*. Flavonoids, simply put, supply the red, orange, and yellow colors found in fruits, vegetables, and almost all other plants. Their therapeutic benefits are vast, making them an important part of natural medicine. Flavonoids' protective and healing repertoire includes helping control blood pressure and fighting inflammation to guard against heart disease, lowering blood sugar to avoid diabetes, protecting cells against cancer invasion, and keeping brain cells strong to fight dementia. For centuries, polyphenols have been a key part of traditional Ayurvedic and Chinese medicine for these reasons and more.

Chlorophyll

Chlorophyll is responsible for the green color in cannabis and many other plants. It is filled with phytonutrients. While not deemed essential for human health, it helps detoxify the body, boosts energy, supports the immune system and the transmission of impulses through nerves, and helps with muscle relaxation.

Terpenes

Terpenes (a word often used interchangeably with *terpenoids*, which are terpenes that have undergone oxidation) are known for their unmistakable scents, such as pine, menthol, cinnamon, and cloves, to name a few. They are also known for their colors—think the red of a tomato or a sunflower's brilliant yellow. They give their host plants (and some insects) some of their unique characteristics, which we are able to enjoy through our senses. For instance, from an aromatherapy standpoint we may link the unmistakable scents that come from terpenes found in evergreen and eucalyptus to uplifting or relaxing experiences.

But terpenes also have an internal, biological effect when ingested. The therapeutic benefits of terpenes have been acknowledged and recorded since the advent of written texts. From the taste of a fruit to the succulent scent of a tree, terpenes interact with receptors in the brain. They may, for instance, enhance dopamine activity, which creates a feeling of pleasure, or work similarly to a serotonin reuptake inhibitor (SSRI), a type of prescription anti-depressant that increases serotonin levels.

When I suggested at the beginning of this chapter that your experience with CBD will likely happen in conjunction with other biological components in plants, I was largely talking about terpenes. Holistic health practitioner and herbalist Rachelle Robinett explains, "Terpenes are largely responsible for how and why certain herbs are considered allies' for CBD—from increasing the efficacy of CBD to working on the endocannabinoid system, providing complementary benefits, and more." This idea will come up again when we talk about the interaction of whole-plant cannabis in the endocannabinoid system.

Though there's not enough room to go into all the terpenes here, I think it is helpful to understand how a few of them work. You might see individual terpenes can be listed on cannabis-product labels because they contribute to the CBD experience. Beta-caryophyllene is a terpene found in cannabis as well as basil, oregano, and black pepper. In 2008, the Swiss scientist Jürg Gertsch documented beta-caryophyllene as "a dietary cannabinoid," meaning it is consumed like a food. It is recognized as the only terpene to directly activate cannabinoid receptors (which we will learn about in the next section).

Another important terpene is D-limonene. As you may suspect from the name, it is found in the peels of limes, lemons, and other citrus fruits. Its refreshing scent can have an uplifting effect, and it has the ability to help reduce anxiety and stress. It is also recognized as an anti-inflammatory and antioxidant and can decrease blood sugar and blood pressure.

Cannabinoids

Cannabinoids are a diverse subclass of terpenes and a diverse class of compounds found in cannabis and other plants, including cacao, black pepper, echinacea, and more. Cannabinoids deliver the beautiful healing properties we hear so much about in cannabis. While all varieties of cannabis have cannabinoids, specific combinations of cannabinoids are unique to different strains of cannabis. There are over one hundred different cannabinoids, several of which have been researched but to date the majority have not. The most familiar are CBD and THC, although our knowledge of even these is limited because the long-time illegal status of cannabis has prevented scientists from researching them further.

CBD, a nonpsychoactive compound, is the most widely researched of the cannabinoids; it is recognized as an analgesic, anti-inflammatory, antioxidant, and a neuroprotectant (meaning it can help fight or protect against neurodegenerative disorders by boosting brain cell production). THC, a psychoactive compound, is becoming increasingly recognized for its medicinal applications. THC, like CBD, is an analgesic, anti-inflammatory, antioxidant, a neuroprotectant, and it also has muscle-relaxant properties.

THE ENTOURAGE EFFECT

While it's good to know what some of the compounds in cannabis do by themselves, research suggests that these compounds may provide additional benefits when they act together. This synergy between cannabis compounds has been coined the "entourage effect." The term was first used in the context of cannabis in 1998 by Israeli organic chemist and professor of medicine Raphael Mechoulam in a paper called "Taming THC: Potential Cannabis Synergy and Phytocannabinoid-Terpenoid Entourage Effects." What does the entourage effect mean for CBD? Whereas CBD by itself targets very specific functions in the body, CBD in its whole-plant cannabis form may address many more functions in the body, providing a variety of benefits that are delivered to all parts of the body, thus helping it achieve or maintain balance. Entourage effect aside, that healing synergy can come not just from the components *within* a single plant, but also from combined components *between* two different kinds of plants—such as when cannabis and echinacea or cannabis and chamomile are used together.

The entourage effect suggests that CBD could prove more beneficial when joined by flavonoids, terpenes, and other natural components found throughout the cannabis plant. That's why you might hear recommendations to use CBD products that include all parts of the cannabis plant—flowers, leaves, stems, and roots. It's so you get the benefit of the compounds from every part of the plant. Such products use full-spectrum extracts, which we'll learn more about in chapter 3.

Research on the exact ways in which the entourage effect works in the body is preliminary, as opportunities to study it more closely have been limited. It is worth noting that there are potential downsides to consuming a CBD product made from the whole plant. Different cannabinoids act on several different receptors in the human body at the same time. While some compounds may be helpful for treating a condition or achieving a certain state of being, others may have undesirable effects or are at least not necessary to achieve the effects you want. In fact, some cannabinoids can invoke effects that are the complete opposite of the desired result. Essentially, whole-plant consumption throws an unknown and unquantified combination of cannabinoids at the receptors in your body.

Additionally, products infused with whole-plant extracts may deliver inconsistent results because each plant, even from the same strain, is unique and will have a slightly different combination of compounds. A report in *Nature* from 2018 found that the cannabinoid content of legal cannabis in Washington state varies across consumer products and even across testing facilities.

I don't believe that either extreme—whole-plant consumption or isolate consumption—is ideal. Further scientific research is needed to determine the facts around proposed theories, facts that can advise on product formulations so they can be made with scientifically backed, reliable, and consistent effects. For now, if you are looking to support your endocannabinoid system and attain or maintain balance, full- and broad-spectrum CBD products (described on page 59) are a good starting point. If you are seeking to target a particular condition, look for specific combinations of plant molecules from cannabis or complementary ingredients. For instance, if you are looking for an uplifting sublingual (something taken under the tongue), find a full- or broad-spectrum product that has higher concentrations of energizing terpenes like limonene and myrcene or a product made from a CBD isolate containing complementary ingredients like terpenes or foods and spices such as citrus fruits, cinnamon, and clove.

THE ENDOCANNABINOID SYSTEM

Now that you know about the beneficial compounds in cannabis, it's important to understand how they work in our bodies. The human body has a little-known system that produces and uses molecules like those the cannabis plant produces. In fact, in the 1990s, when the system was discovered, it was named for the cannabis plant: the endocannabinoid system, or ECS.

Researchers have found that the main function of this system is to impart homeostasis, or balance, to the body. That means the ECS helps keep the body's most vital systems functioning in a beautifully balanced way, from the heart to the lungs, the gastrointestinal tract to the brain, and on to the immune system. It's "one of the most important physiologic systems involved in establishing and maintaining human health," notes Dr. Bradley Alger, one of the most widely published researchers studying endocannabinoids in the brain. He explains that the ECS is comprised of "endocannabinoids and their receptors [which are] found throughout the body: in the brain, organs, connective tissues, glands, and immune cells." This widespread network also includes a third component, proteins called enzymes that help produce and break down endocannabinoids. Together, these three components comprise the ECS, keeping the body functioning and in balance and helping it return to health when imbalance, or disease, takes hold.

The ECS may even play a special part in mind-body healing. Dr. Alger notes: "With their complex actions in our immune system, nervous system, and virtually all of the body's organs, the endocannabinoids are literally a bridge between body and mind. By understanding the endocannabinoid system, we begin to see a mechanism that could connect brain activity and states of physical health and disease."

ECS Receptors

Throughout the ECS, a series of receptors attached to cell membranes monitor messages between cells in order to keep bodily processes running smoothly. The two most prominent are cannabinoid receptors 1 and 2, or CB1 and CB2. CB1 receptors are largely found in the central nervous system, including the brain, spinal cord, and nerves. CB2 receptors line the immune system, including the lymph nodes and bone marrow. Receptors can also be found in organs, such as the liver and spleen; muscles; connective and fat tissues; and glands. As long as these receptors are messaging smoothly, all is well. When even a slight hiccup occurs, our bodies naturally produce endocannabinoid molecules to interact with the receptors to get messaging back on track.

Endocannabinoid Molecules

Endocannabinoid molecules work by interacting with receptors. Technically speaking, endocannabinoids are neurotransmitters produced inside our bodies. *Endo* is the Latin term for "internal." They come to the rescue when receptors are not signally correctly and help them return to normal. As you learned above, cannabinoids also exist outside our bodies, usually in plants. If the body for some reason cannot produce enough endocannabinoids when a receptor needs them to help keep systems humming, those outside cannabinoids become useful. They can be delivered though the foods and nutrients we consume. The ECS is designed to receive all cannabinoids, whether internal or external. They can also be stimulated through the terpenes and flavonoids that accompany the cannabinoids in the aforementioned foods and spices, and in the complementary ingredients in the recipes in chapter 5.

Enzymes

Enzymes are a vital part of the ECS as they both build and break down endocannabinoids in our bodies. Some enzymes synthesize the endocannabinoids anandamide and 2-AG (2-arachidonoylglycerol) using the fat in our bodies. Other enzymes take the form of transport proteins specific to the ECS. When our internal operating systems require endocannabinoids, these enzymes spring into action. Because endocannabinoids are fat-soluble and our bodies are comprised of water, these enzymes help move endocannabinoid molecules throughout the body. The two enzymes that are widely studied across the ECS are FAAH (fatty acid amidohydrolase) and MAGL (monoacylglycerol lipase); FAAH is responsible for breaking down anandamide and works in tandem with MAGL to break down 2-AG. The creation and breakdown of endocannabinoids happens "on demand" when smooth communications between receptors deteriorate. As communications become smooth again, the endocannabinoids are then broken down by enzymes, and the body returns to business as usual.

HOW DOES CBD INTERACT WITH THE ECS?

Whether consumed internally or applied topically, CBD has an indirect effect on the endocannabinoid system. The CB1 receptor—predominantly found in the brain and nervous system—and the CB2 receptor, found throughout the immune system and other operating systems of the body—interact in different ways with different cannabinoids. While THC is known to bind with both receptors, CBD does not. CBD does, however, interact with these receptors. For instance, it can prevent THC from binding with CB1 receptors, thus minimizing its psychotropic effects and potentially decreasing anxiety and any potential memory impairment associated with THC use.

In addition, CBD is known to bind and otherwise interact with other receptors throughout the body—in the nervous system and elsewhere—for beneficial effects. Experiments have shown CBD to have neuroprotective, anti-inflammatory, and analgesic properties. It can also help increase the number of endocannabinoids our bodies naturally produced. It also has a direct effect on receptors in other parts of the body, including non-cannabinoid receptors that make up our behavior and cognitive centers for motivation and reward such as opioid receptors, pain regulation receptors, dopamine receptors, and serotonin receptors, which affect depression and anxiety.

When applied topically, CBD interacts with receptors in skin to reduce pain and inflammation. Trista Okel, founder of Empower Body Care, explains that CBD is "particularly helpful as an antinociceptive, which means that it 'turns down the volume' of the pain signal by reducing the central nervous system's response to painful stimuli." CBD also suppresses the production of inflammatory enzymes in the skin and activates the PPAR-y receptor, which Trista says "regulates cell life, which includes the regulation of inflammation."

CBD'S POTENTIAL BENEFITS

With this basic information under your belt, it's time to start thinking about how cannabis might work for you. First, it's good to know that cannabis, and specifically CBD, is being widely researched and tested, although it is still a relatively new field, and most of the science behind the biological workings currently lies in animal studies. That's why you will see personal anecdotes in addition to specific research results about CBD's uses and benefits later in this chapter.

Before we get to that, let's review what happens to our bodies when we engage with CBD. The three lists below give a succinct summary of CBD's benefits.

CBD is recognized as an:
- Anti-inflammatory—ramps up the body's defense system
- Antioxidant/neuroprotective—reduces toxicity from external factors
- Antipsychotic—regulates mood, thinking, and perception
- Antimicrobial—kills bacteria (think infection)
- Analgesic—manages pain

Internal effects of CBD:
- Increased relaxation; less tension and muscle stress
- Better sleep and deeper rest
- Diminished anxiety
- Balance of bodily systems including mood and digestion
- Pain reduction through decreasing inflammation

Topical effects of CBD:
- Reduced inflammation, irritation, redness, and bruising
- Increased moisture retention
- Tonal and textural balancing of the skin

CBD AND HEALTH CONDITIONS

The number of ailments that CBD can address seems surprisingly long, even to me. I often find myself amazed at how many conditions it targets. However, if you think about how the endocannabinoid and other response systems work in our bodies and how many ailments, from topical skin conditions to joint pain, are really just inflammation, it makes sense. CBD is an anti-inflammatory, and so it can address an incredible array of ailments, as inflammation is at the core of most conditions from the most minor to some of the most serious.

While CBD has shown potential to positively impact a far greater number of conditions than I cover in this chapter—including neurodegenerative diseases, epilepsy, cancer, and others—I chose to examine the most-common and -discussed ailments. In fact, three of the conditions I'll cover—anxiety, pain, and sleep problems—are the leading conditions affecting Americans. I will also go over the ailments that my peers in the cannabis industry mention most frequently and explore the ways that CBD can impact your quality of life, even if you don't have a serious health condition.

I will share what we know about CBD's effects on your health, alongside stories from experts and advocates in the cannabis and wellness worlds, who have offered their personal experiences with CBD's therapeutic properties. I hope that these stories will give you the confidence to explore CBD and consider how it can relate to your experiences with your body.

Anxiety, Stress, and Depression

Stress, depression, and anxiety are not just trending topics but conditions that affect a staggering number of people. In fact, a staggering 40 million adults in the United States alone suffer from an anxiety disorder. *Anxiety* has become a buzzword these days, used to describe a range of feelings. For some, it means that they have too much on their plate, which has created a sensation of unease and worry; for others, it characterizes a nervous disorder with compulsive behavior. The *Diagnostic and Statistical Manual of Mental Disorders* (*DSM-5*) describes one of the criteria for a diagnosis of generalized anxiety disorder as "excessive anxiety and worry (apprehensive expectation), occurring more days than not for at least six months, about a number of events or activities (such as work or school performance)." Anxiety can manifest in various physical symptoms, from sweating and shortness of breath to panic attacks.

Stress is similarly defined as tension and mental or emotional strain caused by similar brain signaling. Physical symptoms manifest in diverse ways—including headaches, insomnia, and muscle tension—while emotional symptoms include mood swings, anxiety, and a feeling of overwhelm. Furthermore, stress, according to the staff of the Mayo Clinic, can contribute to more serious health conditions, such as high blood pressure, heart disease, obesity, and diabetes, so it is imperative to manage and, if possible, eliminate its contributing causes.

The state of depression is characterized by persistent feelings of sadness that result in changes in sleep, self-esteem, appetite, moods, and more. Clinical depression is thought to result from a chemical imbalance; however, the causes are more complex and diverse than that, ranging from genetic predisposition to lifestyle factors. In fact, life's stressors, such as the loss of a loved one or a job change, could trigger the onset of depression for some people.

CBD activates cannabinoid and other receptors that give you feelings of pleasure and encourage the production of mood-boosting neurotransmitters. It interacts with serotonin receptors in the brain,

CBD AND ANXIETY

Licensed clinical social worker Lauren Passoff shares her personal experience with CBD, stress, and anxiety.

> I had my first bout with anxiety at twenty-two, when I was walking down the street and for no "apparent" reason, I felt anxious. This was not [normal stress]. This was a feeling of "impending doom" that was exacerbated by not understanding why or where it was coming from. . . . The perpetual fear that this could happen again anywhere at any time, and again for no plausible reason . . . began a cycle of anxiety that has consistently reared its ugly head throughout my life. . . .
>
> I had to learn and accept that [anxiety] may be a part of the complex yet wonderful persona that is me, and it became imperative that I learn more about it, increase my self-awareness, and learn what to do when these feelings of anxiety left me in what felt like a debilitated state. This is where CBD comes in. I had a friend, a fellow social worker, recommend it to me, and ever since then, it is both a preventive measure and coping strategy that I use to manage and satiate my ugly friend anxiety. Due to the quick onset time of anxiety and panic attacks, I like to have CBD flower available for inhalation. There are some great vaporizers on the market now that provide just that. I also pre-roll botanical blends of CBD flower and other herbs for a balanced experience.

boosting the signaling of neurotransmitters to enhance mood. A study published by the National Institutes of Health's National Library of Medicine acknowledges the antidepressant-like effects of CBD in rodents and found that CBD has synergistic effects when it is administered with antidepressants. Some CBD products also contain other mood-boosting compounds found in the cannabis plant, such as D-limonene, a terpene with mood-elevating properties that was discussed earlier in this chapter. A study in which limonene was inhaled by mice showed that it potentially reduced their anxiety.

CBD also inhibits the production of the FAAH enzyme described earlier in this chapter. Reduced FAAH enzyme levels may increase endocannabinoid signaling and levels of anandamide, an endocannabinoid that regulates pain and moods, and controls inflammation. (Its name comes from the Sanskrit word *ananda*, meaning "joy" or "bliss.") It also may decrease "threat-related amygdala reactivity," meaning one would experience diminished emotional reactions to threatening experiences, according to one study that examined the gene affecting FAAH production in healthy adults. Simply having the gene that reduces FAAH levels can make someone less vulnerable to developing anxiety-related symptoms. CBD, which increases anandamide in the body by inhibiting the FAAH enzyme, could have a similar impact.

Pain

Pain is a huge issue for many people around the world. It is, in fact, one of the largest market segments for cannabis product sales to date. The Centers for Disease Control and Prevention (CDC) reported that approximately 20 percent of the US's adult population suffers from chronic pain, with about 20 million of those people experiencing limitations in their daily activities because of it.

The origins of pain are so diverse that it makes it difficult to speak about its causes in brief, but it is important to address the two different forms of pain: acute and chronic. Acute is the type of pain that has a sudden onset with a clear cause—think a bonk on the knee or twisted ankle—and chronic pain is a persistent feeling of discomfort caused by an underlying condition.

There are a couple of theories that speak to the effect of cannabis on pain. It has been widely discussed that the combination of THC with CBD is important for maximum relief. One reason for this is that THC, unlike CBD, stimulates neural pathways and interacts with the brain on a neuropathic level, which directly affects the pain response that is coming from the brain. CBD on its own, though, can still be effective for pain management.

In one study, researchers found that CBD reduced pain by interacting with serotonin receptors, which affect your body's pain response, but its effect on the nerves themselves is yet unknown. Another study showed that CBD belongs to a class of cannabinoids that can reduce neuropathic pain by targeting glycine receptors (GlyRs) in the central nervous system. GlyRs are believed to mediate the sensation of pain in the body. Studies conducted on rats have also shown that repeated low doses of CBD can have a pain-relieving effect.

Preliminary research indicates that CBD reduces inflammation, which in turn reduces pain. Dr. Sota Omoigui, a medical director of the LA Pain Clinic, says, "Irrespective of the type of pain, whether it is acute or chronic pain, peripheral or central pain, nociceptive or neuropathic pain, the underlying origin is inflammation and the inflammatory response." He considers an outcome in pain management successful if it leads to less inflammation, regardless if that inflammation comes from arthritis, back and neck pain, fibromyalgia, nerve or neuropathic pain syndromes, migraines, sports injuries, tendonitis, or any other condition.

CBD AND PSORIATIC ARTHRITIS

Boris Shcharansky, COO of Papa & Barkley, a California-based topicals company, describes his personal journey from pain to relief.

My discovery process began when I was diagnosed with psoriatic arthritis in late 2011 after experiencing some severe inflammation in my toes, ankles, and lower back. I visited a rheumatologist, who gave me a choice of either methotrexate or sulfasalazine, both immunosuppressant drugs used in early-stage cancer treatments. They each came with a list of side effects, with the most extreme being a "potential" risk of deformities in your children. Although there were other, very concerning side effects listed (sudden death, cancer, [and] tuberculosis, to name a few), this was the one that my wife paid the most attention to once I got home. I was in so much pain at the time—my work took me around the world for various meetings, and I was logging over one hundred thousand miles annually. The constant stress on my body pushed me to the edge, and I was ready to take anything they threw at me. Luckily, I have an amazing wife who is not as reactive as I am. She threw away the pills, and we started exploring alternative treatments. On a trip to California, I was introduced to the Cannatonic strain of cannabis, which has a flower with 2:1 ratio of CBD and THC. After two days of just smoking this flower, my inflammation was gone from my feet, ankles, and back. Since then, I have moved on to capsules and tinctures for my CBD ingestion, and I have been able to return to playing tennis and road biking, tasks which I thought were closed to me since my diagnosis.

To address both acute and chronic pain with CBD, it is important to identify the proper dose and dosing methods to experience the benefits (see page 62 for further details). For those experiencing chronic pain, CBD can be used not only to tackle the immediate sensation of pain but also to manage the pain if a consistent level of CBD is maintained in the body for an extended period of time. As mentioned above, THC may also be an important component in your cannabis product because chronic pain often has a neurological component. For acute pain, such as the pain often associated with an injury, it is valuable to use a CBD product that has immediate onset and continues to have effect for as long as the pain lasts. I suggest starting with a smokable and then consuming an edible that has a delayed onset but will last for a longer duration.

Gut Health

The gut is an essential part of the body, not only helping us digest food and remove waste but also serving as the home of our microbiome. Our microbiomes have been found to affect our immune system, metabolism, mood, sleep, and even our behavior.

The gut contains endocannabinoid receptors, including CB1 and CB2. Dr. Mollie Parker Szybala, a naturopathic doctor of Sun Valley Natural Medicine and a specialist in the microbiome, explains these receptors in the gut "function to regulate GI movement, hunger, inflammation, how the gut and brain communicate, and help maintain the integrity of the gut lining. To maintain wellness in the gut, we must have proper endocannabinoid tone, which means the CB1 and CB2 receptor activity is well balanced. When out of balance, the gut lining can break down, allowing for harmful substances to pass from the gut into the bloodstream, causing a condition called leaky gut." She notes,

"Proper endocannabinoid tone has also been shown to modulate the gut microbiome, increasing beneficial bacteria and reducing harmful bacteria." CBD can help by delivering cannabinoids the body needs to achieve proper endocannabinoid tone.

CBD's value as an anti-inflammatory can help the gut as well. Leaky gut ultimately creates inflammation leading to issues not only in the digestive tract but also in the bloodstream. According to Dr. Marcelo Campos, a contributor to Harvard Health Publishing, current research shows "modifications in the intestinal bacteria and inflammation may play a role in the development of several common chronic diseases," including Crohn's disease, chronic fatigue syndrome, obesity, and certain kinds of mental illness. In fact, much of the medical community believes that we all suffer from leaky gut to one degree or another due to stress and our modern diets, which tend to be high in sugar.

Beauty and Skincare

Beauty truly does start on the inside, and it is more than a look—it is a state of being. Looking good is possible only if you do actually feel good physically. They go hand in hand. Tension in the body can appear as a furrow in your brow, and an imbalanced digestive system can produce extra oil on the skin. In talking about beauty and skincare, we need to address both the topical and the internal.

As nutrition rises to the forefront of our considerations for health and wellness, so does the movement for addressing skin health from the inside out. It is no secret that skin is our largest external organ. It is the exterior piece of an intricate operating system that not only holds the body together, but also reflects what is happening on the inside. While foreign objects, air pollution, and free radicals affect our skin from the outside, our skin supports our insides by acting as a barrier to

CBD AND GI ISSUES

Dr. Mollie Parker Szybala has had personal experience with CBD and its effects on her digestive health.

There was a period of time in my life when I would hesitate, in a moment of panic, before eating a meal, never knowing how it would make me feel or if it would cause me any harm. I feared going out to eat or going to dinner parties with friends. Every day was a struggle knowing that I would be dealing with varying degrees of fatigue, discomfort, and anxiety with no end in sight.

Growing up with chronic GI issues was a challenge, as I was constantly looking for anything to help improve my overall health and well-being. I remember seeing doctor after doctor, all of whom had suggestions for different prescriptions that would help relieve some of my symptoms but never provided a root-cause treatment that would lead to long-term health.

When conventional therapies did not allow me to achieve my health and wellness goals, I began seeking out alternative treatments. It wasn't until I saw a naturopathic physician that I finally felt like my symptoms were validated and realized the power I held to improve my own quality of life. I was diagnosed a celiac. I learned about the benefits of gut-healing foods and specific nutrients I could seek out to improve my quality of life.

I use CBD to assist in healing leaky gut, improve the well-being of my microbiome, and reduce inflammation. It also provides me a sense of calm, lessens anxiety, and allows me to get rest necessary to heal. Food is a form of medicine, and I love feeling empowered when I am able to incorporate healing herbs, like CBD, into my meals to take control of my health.

the external forces. Skin is also our first indicator of stress in the body. Ayurveda and Chinese medicine have long since looked at the skin to determine what is going on internally.

Addressing the simplest of imbalances with a daily CBD supplement is an opportunity to bring your skin one step closer to the coloration and texture you want. I take about 10–30 milligrams of CBD daily when I am not addressing anything specific and just want to balance my system; I have to say that my skin is far clearer and even-toned for it. After taking three years of daily doses of CBD oil under my tongue or added to a beverage, I am less inclined to wear lots of makeup or feel the need to "prepare" my skin for the day.

CBD is, as you know, an anti-inflammatory, and many skin conditions are caused by inflammation. Internal conditions caused by inflammation manifest on the skin as well. Think about sleep deprivation resulting in bags and purple circles under your eyes. Relax your mind and calm your stress and the furrow in your brow disappears. That said, there are topical remedies with CBD available that address inflammation on a superficial level as opposed to a systemic level. They can smooth puffiness and fine lines by reducing topical inflammation.

Exercise Recovery and Performance

Though largely studied as a tool for pain management and mitigation, CBD has been shown in some trials to enhance exercise performance and recovery.

Dr. Alan Beyer, a sports medicine doctor and an executive medical director of the Hoag Orthopedic Institute in California, explains in a *U.S. News & World Report* article, "Any workout, especially a rigorous one, causes microscopic damage to the body's muscles and tissues. . . . [T]oo

CBD AND SKINCARE

During early testing of Verté Essentials' topical beauty products, I was introduced to the fabulous Carla Butts, a licensed master esthetician with twenty years of experience. Here, she speaks about her experience with CBD skincare.

> I became interested in CBD as a co-therapy with cold-extracted botanicals, vitamins, minerals, peptides, and human-derived stem cell technology when I was given access to a unique form of nanoparticulated CBD that is water-soluble and penetrates the skin with incredible efficiency. Not only did I see the natural healing effects of CBD on the skin, but in tiny molecular form [it] increased the efficacy of other natural ingredients used in concert.
>
> With something this powerful, less can be more. Initial use can temporarily drive issues to the surface, but over time, adding CBD to an existing routine takes the skin to the next level of radiance [and causes a] reduction in redness and irritation, and a seeming reduction in acne lesions. Clients also report additional calmness, general health, and well-being.

much inflammation left unchecked can contribute to excessive muscle damage and poor workout results." CBD helps support faster recovery by mitigating this inflammatory response.

CBD AND PAIN MANAGEMENT

In my experience with developing topicals, I have had the opportunity to work with a number of professional athletes. One of my greatest joys from this process was seeing CBD's success with treating the pain of athletes working at their highest potential physical capacities.

Joey Sides is one of these athletes. He grew up in the outdoors and amidst athletics his whole life, eventually going on to play professional hockey in the US, the Netherlands, and the UK. Throughout his career, he has made all-star teams and served as captain on team after team.

I met Sides in off-season training. He had just been injured, but he was already no stranger to pain, having had an array of injuries, ranging from AC separation to injuries to his ankle and shoulder that required several surgeries.

He reported, "When I strained my quad, I tried ibuprofen, ice, stim units, et cetera, but recovery was still slow. Once I added CBD to my routine, the pain and swelling went down significantly and quickly, so I was able to get back to training and perform on the ice." Reducing inflammation and pain was imperative for him so he could exercise and train the rest of his body, but it also helped prevent further injury by supporting the areas that needed a little more time to heal. As any one of us knows, an injured toe can lead to a weak ankle and affect your gait. Joey's CBD regime allowed him to continue to perform and to improve, allowing him to play on the professional level for another year.

Joey is not the only one. Dr. Amanda Reiman, whose dissertation, "Cannabis Care," was the first study to focus on how medical marijuana dispensaries operate as health-service providers, has conducted research on drug-purchasing behaviors, alcohol-control policies, and medical-cannabis use. She discovered the therapeutic benefits of cannabis when she was young: "I've been an athlete my entire life; from tennis to baseball, cheerleading to gymnastics, my body was giving its all on a regular basis. When I

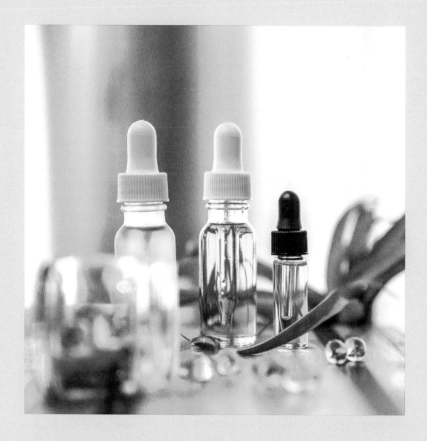

entered my twenties, I began noticing a dull pain after being on my feet for a while. I brushed it off, but it got worse. When I could no longer stand on my tiptoes, I went to the doctor and was told I had osteoarthritis in my feet. My doctor offered up a regime of cortisone shots and anti-inflammatories, but I was concerned about the long-term impacts on my body; I wanted to find a better way. I found that in alternative treatments such as Pilates, bodywork, and cannabis."

Sexual and Reproductive Health

Reproductive health affects everyone, no matter the person's gender, sexual preference, race, or socioeconomic status. Plus, it is an area of health that can simultaneously affect your physical, social, and psychological well-being. After all, reproductive and sexual health is about not only the absence of disease but also pleasure and comfort. I have met many people who have had positive experiences using a cannabis product for their sexual and reproductive health—be it through ingestible products, topicals, or suppositories.

Many women have experienced some pain or discomfort with their monthly cycle or menopause. Symptoms associated with menstruation include abdominal cramping, spasms, muscle aches, and even nausea and diarrhea. Postmenopausal women may experience hot flashes, mood swings, insomnia, mental fog, depression, headaches, bone loss, and more.

There is a concentration of endocannabinoid receptors in the uterus, but there hasn't been much opportunity to study the effect of cannabis on women's health. However, CBD's demonstrated anti-inflammatory and pain-relieving effects can help target uterine pain and many symptoms of menopause. For example, up to 50 percent of women experience bouts of insomnia due to hot flashes, mood changes, stress, and anxiety for the duration of menopause, which can last between one and ten years. All of these conditions can be addressed with CBD supplementation, as we saw earlier in the cases of anxiety and stress.

There is research that suggests that endocannabinoid deficiencies may play a role in early onset menopause. There may also be a link between endocannabinoid levels and estrogen levels. Reduced levels of estrogen are one source of the symptoms mentioned above. By supplementing the endocannabinoid levels in the body, CBD can potentially stimulate the ovaries and in turn help your body produce more estrogen, helping you regulate imbalances and feel better.

Endocannabinoid receptors have also been found in cells that regulate the male reproductive system. In rodents, the presence of anandamide may impact sperm function. The effects of cannabis on male reproductive health are, however, inconclusive at best, with studies offering conflicting insights. The US National Library of Medicine reviewed the findings of previous studies on cannabis and sperm count and concentration and concluded: "Current research suggests that cannabis may negatively impact male fertility." A study led by the Harvard T. H. Chan School of Health reached the opposite conclusion, linking a higher sperm count to men who had previously smoked cannabis. Further research is needed before we can draw any definitive conclusions.

The need for more research doesn't seem to influence the cannabis industry much, as the market of CBD-infused lubricants has exploded. (Many contain carrier oils that are not compatible with latex, so choose wisely.) These products have been created with the idea that CBD can increase blood flow, which in turn is thought to amplify nerve sensation, increasing sexual pleasure. There has been some research into the potentially positive role that cannabis can play in women's sexual health specifically. A study with more than 373 participants showed that about 7 of 10 women in their studies experience more sexual pleasure when using cannabis, with 60 percent of participants experiencing a boost in their libido. That said, most of our knowledge about the connection between cannabis and sexual health comes from observational studies like this one. Furthermore, there has been less formal research and fewer surveys conducted on the effects of cannabis on men as well as nonbinary individuals.

Sleep

Sleep issues have become a modern-day plague. The causes can be diverse, ranging from genetics to external factors like ambient light and noise. Many people have used CBD as a sleep aid and had great success with it.

Much of the preliminary research on the effects of CBD on sleep has centered around the combination of THC, which has sedative effects, and CBD. One of the most thorough studies was conducted using full-spectrum flowers that contained an average of 20 percent THC (with THC levels not exceeding 30 percent) and all other cannabinoids,

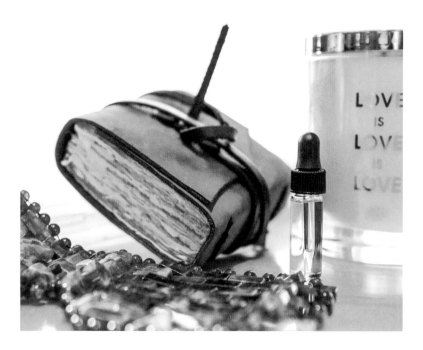

CBD AND BEDTIME ROUTINE

Cannabis advocate Kristen Williams described for me her personal self-care journey and how CBD has enhanced her bedtime routine.

Every night before bed, I moisturize with an all-purpose, CBD-infused balm. After washing my face and changing into my pajamas, I will turn out all the lights except for the little string of lights around my headboard, sit on the edge of my bed, and gently massage this balm to my lips, cuticles, ankles, elbows, and anywhere else that may be feeling like it needs it.

This became an incredibly important ritual for me during college as I juggled classwork, a job, an internship, and trying to launch my own business. I often got too little sleep, and my mind would be racing about what I still had to do and stressing over how tired I would be the next day. When I started this massage routine paired with a nourishing and relaxing balm, I found that I would fall asleep more quickly, sleep more deeply, and wake up feeling refreshed—even when I was operating on only four hours of sleep. Now, after further study of cannabis and other herbs, I better understand and appreciate that the act of self-massage can help boost my endocannabinoid levels, relaxing me and signaling my body that it's time for bed so that I can get truly deep, restful sleep.

including CBD. The results were promising. Participants rated their level of unrest on a scale of 1–10 (10 being the worst), and after smoking the flower, the ratings decreased by about 4.5 points on average. It is difficult, however, to determine which of the cannabinoids or other phytochemicals of the plant contributed to the experience. For example, the terpene myrcene—found in cannabis, mangos, hops, and basil, among other foods—is a great complement or potential alternative to THC due to its own sedative effects.

In the end, it's important to keep in mind that sleeplessness is largely a side effect of many other conditions that can be addressed with CBD. Insomnia is often a symptom of stress, anxiety, and depression, which are in fact the leading causes of sleeplessness. In a recent study, researchers studied a group of seventy-two adults. Every member of the group had anxiety, and twenty-five experienced sleep issues. Administration of CBD led to improvement in sleep in the first month. This study focused on the relationship between sleep and anxiety, so it is possible that the participants' sleep loss was in part due to anxiety and CBD helped the patients sleep by mitigating that anxiety.

Overall Wellness

The theory of clinical endocannabinoid deficiency (CED) suggests that an endocannabinoid deficiency may play a role in the onset of many neurodegenerative disorders that involve a deficiency in a particular neurotransmitter, such as Parkinson's disease and Alzheimer's disease. Since the development of the theory in 2001, there have been various studies examining whether treatments that address endocannabinoid deficiency can help with these diseases and maintain overall health. Recent research has also documented statistically significant differences in the levels of anandamide in cerebrospinal fluid between healthy

CBD AS A DAILY SUPPLEMENT

Jennifer Skog, founder of *MJ Lifestyle* magazine, offers her experience with incorporating CBD into her daily routine.

> I have had a long-term romance with this feminine plant [cannabis], but shadowed by my own shame of consumption, like many, I kept her a secret. Looking back, I now see that I was actually self-medicating. As an artist, cannabis helps me release some of the self-doubt and anxieties I have while creating. She allows me to focus on the task at hand and enjoy myself at the same time. Since incorporating CBD tinctures in my daily routine, I feel significantly more grounded and level-headed.

individuals and those who suffer from migraines. Advanced imaging studies have demonstrated adults with post-traumatic stress disorder have a low-functioning ECS.

In addition to maintaining a healthy lifestyle by eating well, exercising, getting enough sleep, and avoiding stress, taking CBD might support your ECS. Studies and clinical data gathered on CED have shown that supplemental cannabinoids offered benefits and relieved symptoms for these disorders by decreasing pain and improving sleep, for example. Improving your endocannabinoid tone, or the overall function of your ECS, can help address all of the conditions described above.

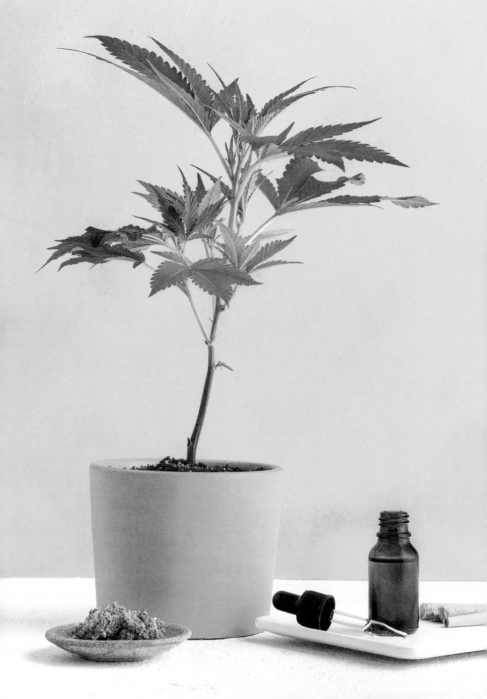

CHAPTER THREE

How to Use CBD

Let's look at CBD as an ingredient and as a standalone product. It comes in a variety of forms—from the whole plant in its natural flowering state to extractions in oils, alcohol, and other solvents, all the way down to an isolate in powder form that can be combined with any number of things. This wide array of options makes CBD perfect for combining with other ingredients in any number of ways.

Today, with the exploding development in the cannabis space, you can get CBD in almost any form you can imagine, from an all-organic raw cacao chocolate bar with honeycomb crystals and chili powder dusted on top to a cold-brewed café latte with natural sweetener. If you can dream it up (and you live in the right location), you can probably find it. CBD can also be infused into foods that are used in cooking, added to beverages, and found in medicinal tinctures and smokables— the list goes on.

To give you a brief overview on what is out there, I'll list the common forms in which you will find CBD and explain how to use them. The amount of CBD in all the products described in this chapter can be found in high and low concentrations—either because the amounts vary in their natural state or simply because the concentrated CBD has been added to a product to meet a certain threshold. (More on how to determine the right concentration and dosage for yourself later.)

CBD FORMS AND METHODS OF USE

Across the regulated and unregulated marketplace, you are going to find a great deal of diversity in the available forms of CBD. The following is a list of the most common forms you will see.

- Capsules and soft gels: contain CBD distillates and extracts, consumed like a traditional supplement
- CBD RSO (Rick Simpson Oil, also called Phoenix Tears): a highly concentrated, dense, liquid form of CBD made from the full plant; has the consistency of honey; dosed in small quantities from a needle-less syringe, consumed sublingually (under the tongue), or as an additive in edibles
- Distillate: made by extracting CBD and other valuable molecules from all the plant matter with an agent such as butane or alcohol and oftentimes found in a carrier oil; designed for inhaling as vapor in a cartridge, vaporizer, or inhaler, or as an additive to another product
- Isolate: the most concentrated, pure form of CBD; the molecule is extracted from the whole plant; has the appearance of yellow to white crystals and can be ground into a fine powder that often does not have an odor or taste; used as an additive
- Oil, extract, and tincture: a liquid form of CBD made from an extraction (or infusion) using the full plant or the addition of a CBD isolate to a base, such as a carrier oil, or, if it is a tincture, alcohol; oils and extracts are consumed sublingually or as an additive to topical products, food, and drink, whereas tinctures are traditionally used exclusively as a sublingual

- Wax and rosin: a highly concentrated solid form of CBD made with resin extracted from the full plant; has a slightly translucent appearance with a texture that can range from gummy to glass-like and comes in shades of green to golden brown; it also comes in the form of shatter (glass-like, transparent extract) and various other products with names that continue to evolve; used for smoking
- Hash and kief: also made from resin, these highly concentrated forms of CBD are made from the small resin glands called trichomes that are found on the cannabis flower and are rich in cannabinoids and terpenes; they are pressed into forms or found loosely in a powdered form; used for smoking or vaping

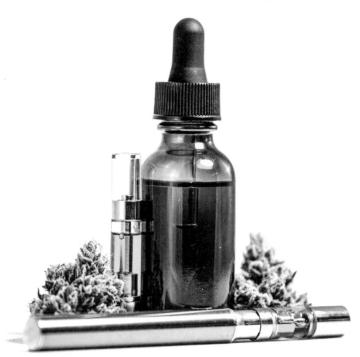

- Whole flower CBD cannabis: cured (dried) CBD-rich cannabis flowers used for smoking, cooking, and for creating extracts

Below are the four types of CBD products explained in order of popularity from what I've seen. Because every person is different, the kind of product that works best for one may not work for another, and everyone must experiment with dosage.

Sublinguals and tinctures: These products are designed to be delivered under the tongue, where the fast-absorbing tissue has quick uptake into the system. This uptake is second to smoking and inhalation for onset speed, but it has none of the side effects. Sublinguals are often found in liquid form, such as oils and tinctures, and will come in a dropper bottle, spray, or pump, with the exception of RSO.

Topicals: A growing category of CBD products, topicals appear in many different forms, from spa and beauty treatments to pain management products. Designed to be applied to the skin to relieve superficial conditions or symptoms, some have deeper penetrating agents that allow for the CBD to move through the skin and into the bloodstream. Most topical products are made from CBD oils and extracts.

Options
- Balms and salves: used for external and superficial skin conditions
- Lotions and oils: used for external skin conditions
- Salts and soaks: used for internal pain relief—CBD is delivered through the skin and into the bloodstream
- Transdermal patches: used for internal pain relief—CBD is delivered through the skin and into the bloodstream

Edibles: The most familiar consumable forms of CBD are food and snack items. They are akin to items you are accustomed to seeing on a grocery store shelf. Their introduction to the marketplace has made cannabis approachable in appearance and easier to consume, as they can mask (or sometimes enhance) the taste of cannabis. When it comes to consumables, I would say there is still a significant shortage of healthy cannabis-infused treats—but, fortunately, we have a chapter full of recipes in this book. When making your own edibles, the oils and alcohol extracts available off the shelf will help you add to and modify most of the recipes' foundational ingredients and guidelines.

Options

- CBD-infused candies, snacks, baked goods, and baking mixes, using different forms of CBD, from extracts to the whole flower, and isolates to RSO
- Fresh CBD-rich cannabis leaves: used for juicing and in smoothies

Inhalants and Smokables: Inhalation and smoking are both done using a variety of apparatuses, from an inhaler to a vape pen to a heatproof bowl that can be used to burn cannabis, releasing smoke for inhalation. Though smoking is the most popular way to consume cannabis in general, smoking and inhalation have not gained the same popularity as delivery methods for CBD, due to the known side effects, namely respiratory issues.

Options

- Smoking: inhaling smoke from whole flower CBD cannabis that is ground up and used in any number of smoking apparatuses from bongs to pipes to rolled in papers; hash, kief, waxes, and resins are also smokable

HEATED OR NOT?

Technically, the cannabinoids in the cannabis plant are in acid form; for example, the precursors to the much-talked-about THC and CBD molecules are tetrahydrocannabinolic acid (THCA) and cannabidiolic acid (CBDA). They do not become THC or CBD, respectively, until we "activate" them by heating them—a process known as *decarboxylation*. The acid forms of these cannabinoids can also be broken down naturally through exposure to air over time, a process called *oxidization*. You should know that most of the products mentioned in this section are produced using CBD, meaning that they have been heated in the extraction or production process. Some of the products you will find are unheated, in which case they will contain CBDA, also known as *raw hemp* or *cannabis*.

The value of this is still being researched fully, but it has been theorized that the unheated form of CBD has a quicker onset and requires less volume for the same therapeutic benefits. The heating process has also been known to kill off active enzymes and terpenes. That said, it is also known to have positive benefits as well. Unlike THCA, THC produces the psychoactive experience. CBD reacts with cannabinoid (and other) receptors to mediate pain, inflammation, and symptoms of disease, while CBDA blocks receptors that cause those conditions, potentially treating the conditions themselves rather than just their symptoms. CBDA is not as stable as in commercial products to date because of oxidization, and it hasn't been studied as readily as CBD, so less information is available as to the benefits. It is hard to recommend one over the other, but ultimately, looking for a full-spectrum product (see page 59) will likely provide the benefits of both CBDA and CBD—at least if you're using it before oxidization has taken place or before you heat the product when you're cooking or vaping it, for instance.

- Dabbing: utilizing a glass apparatus and very high heat from a torch to vaporize the matter into an inhalable state, often done with wax, rosin, and resin
- Vaporizer: inhaling CBD in the form of a vapor, often created by heating cartridges filled with a distillate or an isolate reconstituted with oil; extracts, oils, hash, kief, waxes, rosins, and resins can also be vaped
- Inhaler: inhaling CBD distillate from a pressurized canister or a chamber containing distillate

HOW IS CBD EXTRACTED?

Plants have been used in their extracted forms since ancient times. As a result, there are many different types of extraction methods, many of which are still widely used today in both the home and industrial settings. It's worth taking a look at how CBD products are created for more than a lesson in science. Knowing about them will help you choose one that is best for your body.

The first step for creating any form of CBD is extraction, which involves separating the plant matter containing CBD from the rest of the cannabis plant. Solvent extraction is the most widely used method for creating CBD products at home and commercially. It is the process of dissolving cannabis into a solvent, such as a solution of alcohol, carbon dioxide (CO_2), or butane. Next, any remaining plant matter is strained from the solvent. The solvent is then heated until it evaporates, leaving behind the compounds being extracted.

Some solvents are safer than others. I spoke with Woody Cain, a biochemical engineer, who has coordinated all aspects of quality control in over-the-counter pharmaceutical and cosmetic products for more than seventeen years. While he says that natural ingredients like ether and alcohol, most commonly ethanol, are often used as solvents, they can be flammable and leave toxic by-products. High-level solvent extraction with carbon dioxide, propane, and butane is a common technique, too, but it is complex and expensive, and butane and propane can leave residuals—the safety of which is unknown. Food-grade oils, such as olive oils, can also be used as solvents. Woody recommends them as the most natural and safest options.

As the industry evolves, so will the extraction technology, making products safer for consumption. That has proven to be the case for extractions with solvents like butane and propane on a commercial level. Woody advises to stick to oil-based solvents when you don't know the extraction method used to make a product, and when buying off the shelf, ask for products made with the cleanest new extraction method. (I have always loved solvent extraction with CO_2.)

The substance that is created from extraction is a *full-spectrum* extract of cannabis oil, which contains all of the compounds of the full plant, except the fiber, and includes terpenes, flavonoids, and all the cannabinoids, from CBD to THC and everything in between. A *broad-spectrum* extract is created through distillation, where specific cannabinoids, such as THC, have been removed from a full-spectrum extract. To refine the product even further and separate the CBD, extracts undergo additional processing, thus creating an isolate.

The distinctions between these different forms of CBD and how they are created can be confusing, so let's explore this process using something we already know: an orange. Just as oranges undergo an extraction process to produce orange juice that contains lots of different substances, such as pulp, cannabis can undergo a process that creates a full-spectrum extract that contains many different compounds from the

Products of the Extraction Process

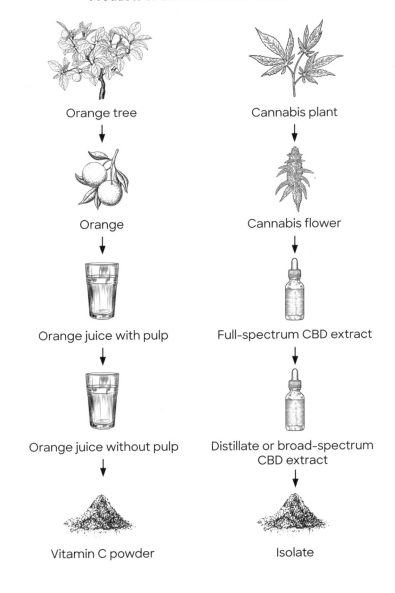

Orange tree

Cannabis plant

Orange

Cannabis flower

Orange juice with pulp

Full-spectrum CBD extract

Orange juice without pulp

Distillate or broad-spectrum CBD extract

Vitamin C powder

Isolate

plant. Before it is packaged into cartons, some orange juice is strained to remove the pulp, as some customers may not want it in their product. Similarly, some full-spectrum extracts can undergo additional processing to remove compounds, such as THC. For those who want the vitamin C from oranges but do not want to drink the juice, the orange can be processed further to produce vitamin C powder. CBD isolates are created with the same idea in mind.

Full-spectrum extracts, broad-spectrum extracts, and isolates are sold in their unaltered forms or combined with other ingredients to create products ranging from topicals to edibles. You will also find two types of products that have undergone additional processing:

A NOTE ON INFUSIONS

You might often see the word *infused* on product labels, but what does this actually mean? I spoke with Olivia Harris, the head of Levo, a company that produces an appliance that helps home cooks easily infuse botanicals into butter and oils. She describes infusions as simply another form of extraction made from soaking plant material in a liquid, such as water, alcohol, or oil. Because many compounds in the cannabis plant, including CBD, are oil-soluble, they do not mix with water. As a result, oil is the liquid of choice for an infusion. Olivia summarizes this concisely: "Infusion is the process of imparting the flavor, nutrients, and aroma of botanicals and herbs into a carrier oil of your choice—from ghee and butter to olive oil, coconut oil, and beyond—using controlled temperature and time."

Nanoparticulated CBD consists of CBD molecules that have been made smaller. Water-soluble CBD is CBD that can be easily mixed with water. Manufacturers suggest that both these products are more easily absorbed by the body, but again, research has not caught up to prove this one way or another. There are many different processes used to create these forms of CBD. Most are patented or considered trade secrets, so both the details of their manufacturing process and the health implications of these processes are unknown.

Choosing the Correct Dose

To date, it has been recognized across state lines within regulated markets that 10 milligrams of CBD is the safe recommended dose. I am 5'2" and 110 pounds, and I have found for my level of moderate activity, diet, and health that taking 7–10 milligrams twice a day has been just the ticket for me to maintain peace of mind. I don't suffer from acute or chronic pain, but I've noticed that taking CBD regularly as a supplement has alleviated a feeling of stress on an ongoing basis. I take this amount using a sublingual, but taking it in any other form will have the same effect for me with a slight variation in the timing (more about this on page 66). I have also noticed, after over three years of regular supplementation, that when I skip my CBD dose for up to two weeks at a time, I still maintain the state of reduced stress that I first noticed when I began taking CBD. This is possibly due to the accumulation of CBD in my system or the balance achieved in my endocannabinoid system. That said, everybody is a different shape and size and processes CBD differently. When you couple this with activity levels, consumption habits, genetics, knowing where to start can be complicated. I hear you, and I'm going to help you out.

Titrating

How do you find that right dose for your body type? It involves a process called titrating. You start with small doses of CBD—or small doses of CBD with a specific combination of ingredients—track how these doses affect you over a specific period of time, and adjust the dosage until you find the perfect amount that works for you. Make sure to titrate with the same product so that you do not introduce any other variables that may throw off your results. Once you find the dose that suits you through titration, you can experiment with different brands or different recipes using the same dose. At this point, if the CBD content of the products are similar, you should require only minor adjustments in the dosage.

Start Small and Dose Up

CBD can take up to three days to integrate into and have an impact on your system, so if at first you are not feeling your intended effects—don't give up. The most important thing to remember is this: The best way to get the best outcome as you integrate plant medicine into your life is to pay attention to how your body reacts. As I said before, everybody is different, and that goes for plants, too.

To start, take the recommended dose of 10 milligrams of your particular product for three days. If you know you are already particularly sensitive to plant medicine, start smaller, with a half dose. If you do not feel any effect after three days of consistent dosing, slowly start to increase your dose, adding another quarter dose to what you are already taking. Try this new dose for three days and repeat this process until you begin noticing changes in your body. You may find it helpful to record your dosing and keep track of its effects in a journal, particularly if you are changing products. Some journals have preprinted templates that give you space to record everything from symptoms, pre-dosing notes, the dose itself, post-dosing notes, and so on.

If you are dosing from products sold from a licensed dispensary in states where the sale of cannabis is regulated, you will be getting consistent and regulated doses of CBD, meaning you can trust the consistency of those products. If you are buying online or in a store that is not a dispensary in a regulated state, there are no guidelines or regulations, so you can't really be sure if the dose that you're receiving is what is being advertised. As a result, look for companies that show test results on the presence of cannabinoids and terpenes for every batch.

Remember, CBD and everything else in any plant, including cannabis, will affect everyone differently. Some people will find that they need 5 milligrams twice a day, and others will need that amount three times a day. All are safe doses, as CBD is not dangerous, unless you have a contraindicated condition or medication. While it's incredibly difficult to overdose on CBD, it is possible that too much could make you sleepy. Some people start to hit that threshold at around 30 milligrams, so if you find that you need to dose up to that point, do it at a time when you know getting tired won't impact your day. You should always have an ongoing conversation with a health-care professional about taking CBD and dosing levels, especially when taking other medications.

Microdosing

When I say start small, the word *microdosing* might come to mind. It is a method of dosing that has been adopted from the arena of psychedelics. Created by the Swiss scientist Dr. Albert Hofmann, it is the practice of consuming very small quantities of psychedelic drugs like mushrooms and LSD. These quantities are not large enough to induce a psychedelic trip but still leave users with some beneficial effects. Those who microdose psychedelics report experiencing a boost in creativity, productivity, and overall brain power.

This dosing practice has made its way to cannabis users, who want to experience THC without the intensity of its psychoactive effects. The same principles can apply to CBD users as well. Though not psychoactive, CBD taken in high doses and in a single sitting can have a sedative effect. If taken in small doses at regular intervals, users can experience its benefits over a longer period of time without the potential sedation.

To experiment with microdosing, first find your total daily dose that you want to use for your particular condition. Then break up that dose into equal portions and administer it at regular intervals throughout the day until you reach your full dose. For example, if your dose was a total of 30 milligrams per day in gummy form, you would instead take a gummy with 10 milligrams of CBD three times a day instead of a single gummy with 30 milligrams. Don't forget to consider the other ingredients in your products and how those might be impacted by breaking up your dose. For instance, if you are taking your CBD in the form of a chocolate edible because you want the added anandamide boost from the chocolate's cacao, make sure the cacao volume is high enough so that the smaller dose can give you the benefits you are seeking.

Microdosing has become increasingly popular among cannabis users for good reason. For those of you more familiar with cannabis consumption, you might scoff at microdosing CBD, but again, CBD affects everyone differently and microdosing might be a good option for some.

Dosing Methods

Beyond dosing, the method you choose to consume CBD will have the most noticeable impact on your experience. The ingestion method that you choose should depend on two factors: the condition you are

ONSET TIMES

Smoking/inhalation = immediate to a few minutes

Sublinguals = immediate to 30 minutes

Edibles/capsules = 30 to 120 minutes, depending on how full your stomach already is, since they are entering through your digestive tract

Topicals = 30 to 45 minutes, making sure to not come into contact with water too soon after application so there is enough time for proper absorption

Transdermal patches = 15 to 30 minutes

addressing, and the immediacy of your reaction to CBD. Here are some general guidelines.

The range of onset times, like most things in this emerging space, is variable because we have not had the proper runway to research it fully. The same is true in exploring the bioavailability of CBD in its diversity of forms. *Bioavailability* refers to the amount of CBD that enters into the body, creating its intended affect. Some consumption methods are said to be more bioavailable than others.

The rise of water-soluble and nanoparticulated CBD is a direct response to theories about our bodies' ability to absorb the molecule. Some think that nanoparticulates are more readily absorbed because they are small enough to penetrate the cell wall. Naysayers suggest that the process of creating CBD in this form creates other nanoparticulated by-products that are then also absorbed through cell walls, potentially having unknown side effects.

Those who favor water-soluble extracts believe that these formations will be more easily available to our bodies for absorption because the composition of our bodies is mostly water. Chemically speaking, however, known processes of creating water-soluble CBD just involve adding lubricating chemicals to the compound so the oil-based cannabis molecules do not bind to one another, creating an appearance of molecular combination. This then also puts our bodies in the position of processing additional potentially unnecessary and harmful ingredients. Other theories suggest that because cannabinoids are lipophilic (fat lovers), administering CBD with fatty substances, such as oils, will help the body absorb it. The majority of brands in the marketplace hold fast to this theory, producing products whose cannabis compounds are in their original fatty form.

The best way to determine the optimal dosing method for yourself is to look at the chart on page 66, pick the onset time that is important for your ritual or condition, consider the form in which you prefer to consume, and explore your dosing threshold. When you consider all these factors together, you will figure out what works for you.

When you consume CBD as a supplement, much like taking a daily vitamin, you may feel very little to nothing. It is when you start addressing particular ailments, especially in higher doses, that you may notice a difference, be it relief from specific symptoms or otherwise.

As you experiment with different dosing methods, you might want to consider timed "layering." For instance, if you're using CBD for pain management and require immediate and longer-term relief, you might choose to inhale a form of CBD and follow that immediately with an edible. Smoking has a very short onset time, whereas an edible takes longer to take effect; by the time the effect of the smoking wears off, the edible will be kicking in. Some brilliant companies are starting to bring time-release products to the market, but we are still quite a way off from consistent dosing in that realm, since tight regulations on cannabis haven't allowed us to conduct research on those products.

MAKING A PURCHASING DECISION

There are so many options as to what kind of CBD products to buy and so many claims as to what CBD can actually do. You will find off-the-shelf cannabis solutions in both grocery stores and regulated dispensaries (on a state-by-state basis) alike. It seems like most brands are trying to bring CBD products into the fold these days, from big-name brands to new artisan and boutique businesses.

To be well informed, you will need to read labels and talk to people in stores and dispensaries, all of whom are operating with their own diverse knowledge base and may offer conflicting information. To add another complication, you will not be able to tell if the CBD you want to purchase is coming from plants with a high concentration of CBD, and it will be hard to know if there are potential by-products from extracts. Thus, it is important to consider many different variables before purchasing your product.

Step 1: You're in Charge

The first step toward using CBD is knowing yourself and making the following considerations.

Why Do You Need CBD?

Know why you are buying and using CBD, no matter if the reason is for a supplement or for a very specific ailment. The "why" will be the single most important aspect to buying the right product and making the right recipe—or at least it will put you on the right track! See chapter 2 for details about ailments and the potential relief that CBD can provide.

What Is the Best Form for You?

Determine the best form of CBD for your intended purposes. Do you want just an extract or do you want a concentrate—or are you intending to use a secondary product created for something specific? Refer back to page 53 to learn what form and concentration are right for you. Onset times for each delivery mechanism (see page 66) are just as important as dosage and CBD volume. Additionally, you can look at the details about the different kinds of extracts and concentrates to see what type of CBD on the cannabis spectrum is best for you—whether it is a full-spectrum product or an isolate.

Step 2: Reading the Label

Transparency is key when it comes to labeling, and the following information should be addressed on the label by the brand. If it's not on the label or packaging, it's likely not a good sign. Essentially, if a brand is proud of what it has done, it will tell you.

CBD Volume

Is the amount of CBD listed? It should be. Generally, CBD content is listed in milligrams (mg). The label should also tell you the milligrams per serving. If it does not, you run the risk of purchasing a hemp oil without any CBD in it. In the unregulated market, hemp oil can be made from the CBD-absent hemp seed.

More isn't always better. A higher concentration of CBD does not always mean that it is more effective or the best quality. Compare the cost of the product with its concentration of CBD. Does a product have a high concentration but is the same or a lower price than most everything else on the market? If so, be wary.

Extraction Method

How was the CBD extracted? While this is becoming less important of a consideration, I personally still have attachments to certain extraction methods. I want the method to have the least amount of negative impact on my body and the environment. And while the industry is cleaning itself up quite a bit from the early days, there are still some concerns about the safety of products made using earlier solvent extraction methods, such as ones that use butane and propane (see page 59). No matter what you ultimately choose, just be sure the label tells you how it was extracted. Again, that means the makers are proud to tell you their process.

Hemp or Cannabis

I am often asked, "Is all CBD the same?" The answer is yes, chemically speaking. CBD from hemp is the same as CBD from cannabis and the same as CBD from another plant that contains the CBD molecule (*plant* being key here, as lab-synthesized CBD is not the same). Remember, CBD is CBD is CBD. Most labels in the national (and international) marketplace will indicate "hemp-derived CBD" or something to that effect. There are two reasons for this: The creators of these products need to reassure consumers that their product contains less than 0.3 percent THC, and they need to use industrial hemp for their product to be in compliance with the US Farm Bill.

Sustainability matters when you are looking at the kind of plant used in your product. Cannabis bioaccumulates, meaning it draws toxins from the soil, and the more plant being processed, the higher the risk for contaminants. Extracting CBD from a plant rich in CBD requires less plant matter, meaning that fewer resources were needed to produce your product and the chance of your product containing contaminating by-products is less.

Ingredients

Are the other ingredients in a CBD product complementary and supporting one another? Or is an ingredient, like artificial flavor or a dye, being used to cover up poor quality in a product? I am in the camp of all-natural ingredients and organic when possible. If you want a grape flavor, look for natural grape juice and natural plant-related colors. I realize brown gummies might not be the best-looking treats, but they are likely the real deal—and healthier. Consider that the makers have the opportunity to use natural colors based on the ingredients, and that level of consideration suggests that they care about their product and their end consumer. After all, their product is designed to get into your bloodstream and impact your body in a healthful way. Keep it clean.

Origin

Where was the CBD in your product grown? The origin of your CBD is important. In this highly unregulated space, your cannabis could be coming from anywhere. Most manufacturers like their plant product to come from the US because there are some basic regulations in place. But there are other countries that produce high-quality plants, and to find their products just requires a bit more knowledge and digging. Again, look to the test results to check for contaminants. Because cannabis bioaccumulates—picks up and cleans toxins out of the soil—we want the cannabis to come from an organic growing spot that minimizes the potential for soil contaminants.

I am a big proponent of organic. In the regulated market in the US, it is mandatory that cannabis is grown organically, free of pesticides. This is not the case in the unregulated market, where pesticides are a potential contaminant. Because cultivated crops have pest problems, it's wise to consider buying only organic in the unregulated national and international markets as well.

Sustainability

Who grew the cannabis? What are their practices, environmentally and from a humanitarian perspective? I presented a great deal of information in this book to outline the current state of the industry and the need to be as considerate as possible in the reintegration of cannabis into consumer culture—not just for the health and safety of the consumer, but for the people growing it and affected by the space where it is grown. I don't think it should be a selling point or a luxury for a company to produce a good product that does a good job taking care of the people making it. That should be mandatory. Consider whether a product is produced locally, uses recyclable packaging, comes from a company that offers fair wages and employs women and minorities, and/or is a member of a community that supports social justice and cannabis reform.

Health Claims

Make sure that any health claims on a label are backed up by documented ingredients, testing, and information about origin. It is illegal for companies to make health claims about their CBD products. Companies find ways around it, such as using specific language in the form of a recommendation, like it "may" aid in sleep. Or they may simply name their product with the word *sleep*. By now, you have learned a great deal in this book about CBD, and that should give you a pretty good sense of what it might be able to do for you. Don't be persuaded by any claims on the label, and be empowered by the information you have acquired here.

Step 3: Checking Test Results

Testing is not mandatory—but it should be. Make sure your products have been tested by a third party and that the result is available to you in the form of a certificate of analysis (COA). Testing is based on the batch you are buying from, and it will analyze for not just cannabinoid content, but the presence of any microbes and other contaminants such as heavy metals and pesticides.

Don't be afraid to ask for test results, as they do not always come with the product or they contain too much info to put on a label. Sometimes test results appear on a secondary product label that has been added with the production and testing of each new batch. If you need to ask, which should be a bit of a turnoff in and of itself, go to a salesperson first. If you need to approach the company, do so as well. This is your health and well-being after all.

Currently, if you are buying from an unregulated, open marketplace—either across state lines, online, or in a store that is not a dispensary in a regulated state—you can't really be sure if a product is what the seller says it is. Remember, a dispensary in a regulated state in the US or a store in a legal country outside the US, is going to have a different take and different guidelines for offering products for sale, and likely the guidelines for offering products for sale will be credible. Internationally, for example, CBD in Canada is sold under federal regulation, which requires detailed guidelines and certain levels of quality for the products. By mid-2020, the European Union will have instituted guidelines to regulate novel foods, allowing the sale of edible CBD with less than 0.2 percent THC. (Vape products are excluded as they require further consideration by the EU.)

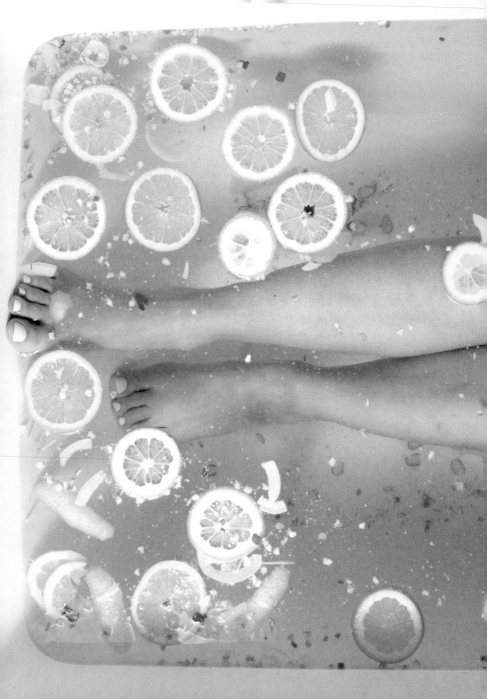

CHAPTER FOUR

Rituals and CBD

DEFINING RITUAL & INTENTION

With the rise in popularity of wellness trends, we hear some words so often that it becomes easy to tune them out. *Ritual* and *intention* are two such words. So, what do they really mean? A ritual involves embracing a process that can naturally invigorate you. Like a habit, a ritual is designed to be repeated. Unlike a habit, it is coupled with joy and intention. Intention is the mental presence and commitment with which you carry out an action. Carrying out something with intention involves deliberation and prudence. Intention is sometimes confused with a goal, the end result of whatever it is you are intending to do, but intention itself is about the path to that goal, the process itself.

When you perform a habit with intention, you turn it into a ritual. The intention and the joy of the ritual are just as important as the result of the ritual itself. The process of developing and performing is, in a sense, how you enjoy the results of your ritual.

Imagine brushing your teeth. As a child, you were told time and time again that you needed to brush your teeth to keep them healthy and strong. Now, after all these years of brushing your teeth, every morning and night you mindlessly walk to the bathroom and retrieve your toothbrush from the holder. You reach for the toothpaste, unscrew the cap, squeeze the commercially prescribed dollop of paste across the bristles, drizzle water on the brush (maybe being careful not to leave the water running), and then you insert the brush into your mouth to scrub around for some time. You are likely looking through yourself in the mirror, mind in another place. Brushing your teeth in this way is an example of a habit.

When I began applying a deeper level of consideration to everything in my life, I found myself shifting my mindset about simple tasks and daily habits, like brushing my teeth, and turning them into rituals. The process of learning what I actually *intended* to get out of the time that I spent brushing my teeth was a gradual progress.

First, I considered why I was brushing my teeth. This reminded me that teeth-brushing is, for me, about preservation, health, and beauty. I considered how I could brush my teeth with only what was needed and nothing more to achieve those goals. I now have a fine-tuned ritual. I put a small amount of tooth powder on my brush as well as my partner's. We then establish a wordless connection in the mirror while we take care of our teeth. The way I brush my teeth today is a reflection of how I am more intentional and invested in every moment of my life.

The act of doing something with deeper levels of consideration and intention has the potential to create a positive impact on you or something around you. Though the word *ritual* implies that those acts are attached to ceremony or something more special than a simple daily habit, you can make the smallest of tasks more profound by completing them with intention and thoughtful consideration. We often try to move quickly toward something we view as an end goal, but if we slow down, we can enjoy the journey as well as the result. Rituals give you more time to embrace life than is often allowed or allotted in our usual time and space.

CBD RITUALS

After you've taken stock of your personal state of well-being and considered the aforementioned applications of CBD, you are probably ready to start creating your own rituals for engaging with CBD. I have included three rituals in this chapter that require nothing except your own body, space, and CBD. Beyond incorporating CBD into your life, the following rituals are also great opportunities to get acquainted with the art of practicing a ritual.

In chapter 5 you will find additional rituals in the form of recipes. The holistic practice of Ayurveda is an example of using recipes as rituals because it honors many plants, including cannabis, as ingredients. It requests that you pay attention to the quality of the ingredient that you choose, what you are doing with an ingredient, and how it makes you feel. This level of consideration is part of the thoughtfulness demanded of a ritual process. Consideration at this level is a form of honoring and caring. By intending to create a nourishing recipe using ingredients that feel good to buy and feel good when you consume them, you have embarked on a ceremonious process. The process continues when you carefully measure out a serving, knowing that this amount is what your body needs and wants; cook and prepare something with love; and consume your creation with that same level of thoughtfulness and gratitude.

Whether you practice one of the rituals in this chapter or make a recipe from the next one, the impetus is intention. The act is ritual. The experience is ceremony.

CBD Meditation

From Michelle Helfner, meditation specialist, acupuncturist, and practitioner of Chinese medicine

Michelle says, "I enjoy my CBD before a meditation, really taking the time to get centered, breathing deeply, and relaxing for a moment first, enjoying it before settling into my meditiation. I noticed adding a ritual designed to increase my well-being [the act of consuming my CBD with intention] has deepened my practice of meditation. Sometimes I take CBD before bed for a more restful night's sleep, which is a meditation in and of itself."

TOOLS

1 dose CBD oil of your choice

Floor cushion or chair (optional)

DIRECTIONS

• Consume your preferred CBD oil. Get into a comfortable seated position. I enjoy sitting on a small cushion, which elevates my seat, crossing my legs in front of me, and resting my hands gently on my knees, with my palms facing upward to the sky. Now, lengthen your spine from your tailbone to the crown of your head.

• Close your eyes. Focus on your breath, noticing every inhale and exhale with a degree of attention to the location of your breath. As you inhale, feel the oxygen glide down the back of your throat and into your chest. Feel it expand your lungs and travel all the way down to your toes. As you exhale, feel the oxygen work its way up from the toes and out of your body, carrying all your thoughts with it, expelling them as it moves. Your breath will clear your mind.

• Let go of all the thoughts that rush through your mind, instead replacing them with your breath. Let go of the need to remember them or write them down. If they are important, they will come back to you. Give yourself a minimum of ten minutes to practice this each day. You may find you can sit in this stillness for only a few moments at a time, and that is OK. Break up the meditation into a couple of shorter sessions throughout the day, if that helps. The duration can and will increase with practice.

RITUAL AND INTENTION WITH CANNABIS

It is important to have context about the relationship between cannabis and ritual and how this history relates to the current pursuit of wellness. My friend, the diversely skilled cannabis professional April Pride, founder of Van der Pop and cofounder of Of Like Minds, offered her voice on the role of ritual and intention in relation to cannabis.

> The sacred status of cannabis has a history on nearly every continent and among cultures that otherwise have conflicting values. From its use to enhance meditation to its purpose within shamanic ceremony, *Cannabis sativa* has had an integral role in intimate, wisdom-seeking ritual since 2500 BCE. The continual use of cannabis is a ritual that has transcended time. Similar to cannabis rituals practiced in each era predating our own, today's rituals are shaped by contemporary materials and technologies. This century's innovations have fueled revolutionary ways to commercialize, consume, and consider this plant. With evermore ways to interact with cannabis, intention determines the products and protocol in cannabis ritual. The ways in which we choose to invest in harvesting intention bring forth very specific tools. Ritual with intention does, in fact, connect through the practice of the ritual itself as well as through the dialogue that it generates.
>
> When modern life has individuals feeling less connected and bombarded with shallow messaging, perhaps this ancient plant provides the blueprint to inspire rituals that can deeply connect us to the divine and greater humanity.

One-Thirds Breath with CBD

From Claudia Nanino, breathwork teacher

Claudia says, "Breathwork is a general term that covers applying control over your breath for a specific amount of time. . . . The breath is the one system of the body that is both voluntary and involuntary, bridging the conscious and unconscious. The beauty of breathwork is that there is no wrong way to do it. You already know how to breathe, and the simple act of being intentional with it brings you into your body and into the present moment." The following exercise is a crowd favorite. "It's simple and effective and when combined with CBD oil, [it] can create a deep sense of calm and relaxation, eliminating stress and anxiety. This simple exercise honors your relationship with your body, the breath, and your inner healer."

TOOLS

1 dose CBD oil of your choice

Floor cushion or chair (optional)

DIRECTIONS

• Consume your preferred CBD oil. Find a comfortable seat either on the floor, a meditation cushion, or a chair. I like to sit on a small cushion, with my legs crossed in front of me, arms outstretched with the back of my palms resting on my thighs, above my knees.

• Make your spine long. Close your eyes. Exhale all of your air. Inhale one-third of your lung capacity, bringing the air into the upper part of your torso and into your lungs. Inhale one-third of your capacity to the middle part of your torso—think about your lower ribs expanding, and breathe into the diaphragm. Inhale the last third of your capacity into your belly.

• Exhale one-third of the air from the belly. Exhale one-third of the air from your middle. Exhale the last third of the air from your upper torso. Repeat at least six times with slow, mindful, continuous inhales and exhales. My practice takes about ten to twenty minutes.

Libby's Moon Ritual

From Libby Cooper, cofounder of Space Coyote

There is a significant number of women who experience discomfort around their moon cycle. This cycle offers the perfect opportunity to explore a self-care practice that uses CBD. Libby says, "Whether your period is light, heavy, regular, or irregular, every woman needs a little support at the end of their cycle. I find this is the perfect time for self-care with a CBD topical rub to ease pain, hydrate, and feel joy. The key to this ritual is finding a CBD topical that you like." While we created this ritual with the female space in mind, anyone can use it for any area of the body that needs a little bit of extra love and attention.

TOOLS

Scented CBD oil or topical CBD rub*

DIRECTIONS

• Wear something long and comfortable, such as a robe. Pour the CBD oil into your hands and rub your hands together, warming up the oil. Take a deep breath, inhaling the scent of the oil. Then massage the warmed oil into your lower abdomen with special focus on your ovaries and uterus both physically and mentally. Repeat on your lower back and inner thighs, making sure to not rush the process.

• Gently lie down in your bed or on your couch. Close your eyes and reflect on how you feel. Slow down your breath and notice how the CBD is starting to relax your muscles and ease tension in your pelvis, which should happen within about two minutes. You may choose to stay here for as long as you like, or you can hop up and continue on with your day once you feel rejuvenated and cramp-free.

*The recipes for CBD Oil (page 92) and Hempsley's CBD-Infused Bedtime Balm (page 132) can be used for this ritual. If using the CBD Oil recipe, add a couple drops of essential oil for a fuller experience.

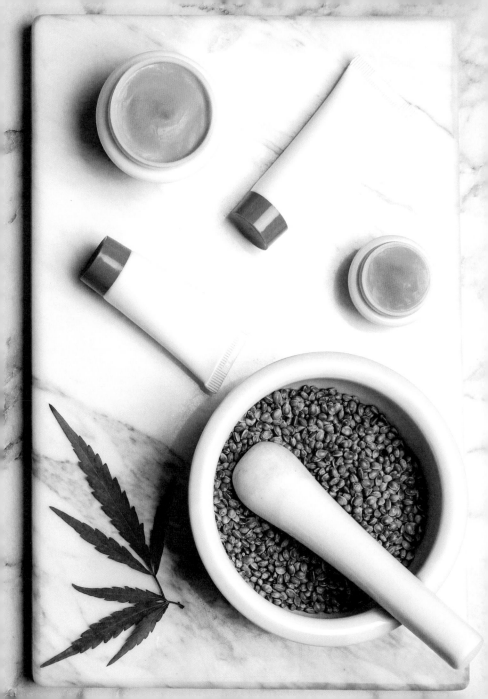

CHAPTER FIVE

CBD Recipes

for the Mind, Body, and Soul

In this chapter, I have compiled a selection of recipes that address some of today's most-talked-about ailments and symptoms. Many of the recipes come from health, wellness, and cannabis experts, who have been gracious enough to share their personal favorites. All of the recipes contained within these pages are designed to be easily prepared in a home kitchen. Additionally, the ingredients are likely available at your local supermarket, and on the occasions when you need some specialty items, I will make a suggestion about where to find them.

Because CBD can be used for a variety of different ailments, I have created a simple key to identify the different applications of each recipe. At the top of each recipe, you will find symbols corresponding to these applications.

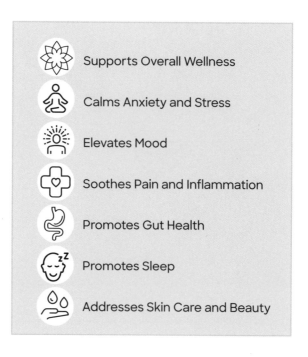

Supports Overall Wellness

Calms Anxiety and Stress

Elevates Mood

Soothes Pain and Inflammation

Promotes Gut Health

Promotes Sleep

Addresses Skin Care and Beauty

Many of the non-CBD ingredients in these recipes are plants that have long been used for their topical and internal healing properties, for everything from inflammation reduction to soothing stomach upset. While CBD is the point of interest here, I'll also touch on the complementary benefits of other ingredients in some recipes, so that you have a thorough understanding of the purpose these ingredients serve, and, in some cases, how they work with CBD.

SOURCING INGREDIENTS

Remember that the efficacy of any recipe is only as potent as everything that goes into it, from the ingredients to the love to the time. Don't skimp. I put a lot of emphasis on the importance of sourcing high-quality CBD earlier in the book, and I hope you keep this in mind as you select the other ingredients that go into these recipes. Remember that any contaminants in your ingredients, such as pesticides or harmful by-products from impure extractions, for example, may adversely affect your body and change the effectiveness of the recipes. Choose products with the best purity, potency, and natural integrity that you can afford. Keep your values close, and don't forget to broaden your considerations (sustainable production, treatment of workers, philanthropy the company engages in) if you have the opportunity to do so. If you need a little refresher on how to make those choices, reference page 73, where we talk about buying considerations for your CBD products.

USING CBD PRODUCTS WITH RECIPES

Preparing your own CBD extracts from scratch for use in foods, snacks, treats, or topicals can be rather complicated, especially in a home kitchen where you don't have access to special lab equipment that measures dosing. Because of this we are not going to address the use of CBD flower in this book, with the exception of one recipe (see Evan's Smoke Blend, page 134). We will simply stick to using CBD oils and extracts that have already been measured for accurate dosing by professionals. Note that each product will have its own recommended dosage guidelines. It is important that you are using the dose that is right for you, because, as we have discussed, every person and every body is different.

When preparing any recipe with CBD extracts, there are a few important tips to keep in mind so that the integrity of your extract is not compromised.

- Never cook items with CBD extracts at temperatures over 245°F (120°C). Never bake them at temperatures over 350°F (175°C). Water boils at 212°F (100°C), so for most recipes, reaching the boiling point means that you are getting too close to a temperature that will compromise your extract.

- For stovetop preparations containing just a few ingredients, add a splash of water to avoid scorching the extracts and creating an awful taste.

- In recipes calling for CBD oil specifically, it is possible to substitute a CBD concentrate or extract. Simply account for the viscosity and the base of your substitute by adding the CBD concentrate or extract to an oil-based ingredient during the heating process to allow for even distribution.

- When choosing a CBD product to add to a balm, make sure that you select one that can be used topically. It should say so on the packaging. Topical dosing recommendations vary dramatically by brand. Expect to see higher doses recommended based on the severity of the condition being addressed. If you're using CBD for routine skin care and supplementation, smaller doses ranging from 2 to 10 milligrams will be adequate.

For the recipe that requires cannabis flowers, it is imperative that you know the flower inside and out before purchasing. The flower should be grown organically with no pesticides, no microbes (think mold), and no heavy metals in the growing medium. You should, in all circumstances, be interested in the CBD levels in the flower. As with readymade CBD products, higher concentrations of CBD in cannabis flowers are not always better; the concentration best for you will depend on the levels of other terpenes and cannabinoids in your flower.

You might be wondering where to purchase that flower. Some countries and some US states still prohibit the sale of CBD hemp flowers, so you may not be able to acquire it on the legal market. For those of you in such states, I hope it is only a matter of time until you have the same access as other places. For those of you in a deregulated state, you can buy online, from a brick-and-mortar retailer that carries it, or from a regulated dispensary. The most reliable source will be the regulated dispensary, as it has more restrictive guidelines on the use of pesticides, the presence of microbes, and the potency and chemical structure (such as the presence of cannabinoids, terpenes, and other content) of the flower. If you buy online or in an unregulated retailer, ask for test results.

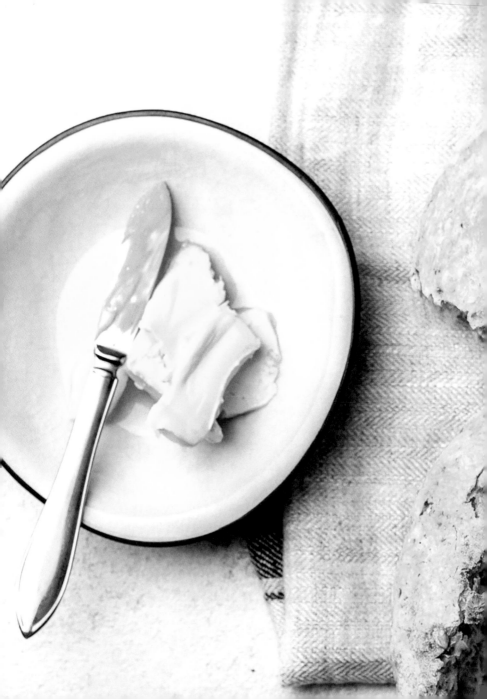

BASIC INFUSIONS

These basic infusion recipes create bases that can be used on their own or in any recipes—for instance, your morning smoothie, a fireside mocktail, or your favorite cookie recipe. The sky is the limit! That said, the recipes in this chapter are tried and true by those who shared them. They are intended to address specific conditions and are suited to do so because of their CBD content, complementary ingredients, and style of ingestion.

You will note that each recipe does not include yields or a specific volume of CBD extract to use to create these bases. That is because you will need to calculate the amount of CBD to use based on the serving size you want. For example, if you are making the CBD Oil and would like 10 milligrams of CBD in 1-tablespoon servings of oil, you will need to do some quick math: one cup of oil has 16 tablespoons, meaning you will need to add sixteen 10-milligram doses of CBD, or 160 milligrams of CBD, in total to achieve your desired results.

Each bottle or package of CBD will let you know how to measure a dose with accuracy. Please use your best judgment when adding your preferred dose of CBD to your recipes. While it has been shown that you cannot overdose on CBD, the incorrect dose might mean that your product won't work therapeutically.

CBD OIL

     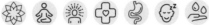

This simple base oil can be used for topical products or cooking.

INGREDIENTS

CBD oil or other oil-based CBD concentrate, such as a shatter or hash

1 cup food grade oil such as MCT (medium-chain triglyceride), coconut, sesame, olive, almond, avocado—the options are limitless

DIRECTIONS

• Combine the two oils in a bowl and whisk thoroughly. If using an oil-based concentrate, combine the two ingredients over low heat, stirring constantly until the CBD concentrate is thoroughly dissolved and mixed in.

• Pour the oil into your storage container. Make sure to shake before using, as the oils may separate after an extended rest period. The shelf life is 2 months if stored unrefrigerated and double that if placed in the fridge.

CBD BUTTER

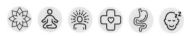

This is simple butter that can be used for any and all cooking and baking. Remember not to let the melted butter go above 350°F (175°C).

INGREDIENTS

1 cup butter

1 cup water

CBD extract

DIRECTIONS

• Add butter and water to a stockpot. Melt the butter on low heat, making sure the water never gets above a simmer. Add the CBD extract while the butter is melting.

• Simmer for 30 minutes, stirring occasionally and thoroughly. Pour the butter into a storage jar. Store refrigerated for up to 2 months. If water forms in the jar, simply drain it off.

CBD HONEY

      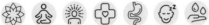

This edible honey can also be used for topical products.

INGREDIENTS

1 cup honey

CBD extract

Water

DIRECTIONS

• Heat the CBD extract and honey in a double boiler, stirring periodically to combine the ingredients. Bring the water to a simmer and maintain for 40 minutes. Pour the honey into a jar. Storing the honey in an opaque jar gives it a shelf life of 2 months.

CBD SIMPLE SYRUP

This syrup can be used as an ingredient in any beverage. You will need coconut-based glycerin for this recipe. To date, it is not something you will find in most groceries, so it's best to acquire it online.

INGREDIENTS

3 cups water

CBD extract

3 cups granulated sugar

3 tablespoons coconut-based vegetable glycerin

Note: If your extract is an oil, use one with a high concentration of CBD so you can use less of it.

DIRECTIONS

• Heat the water in a stockpot on low, so that it never gets above a simmer. Add the CBD extract and stir. Add the sugar, stirring as it dissolves. Simmer for 40 minutes covered, stirring occasionally. Uncover and add the glycerin, stirring constantly for another 5–10 minutes until the mixture thickens. Allow it to cool slightly, and transfer it to a storage container. Store in the fridge for up to 2 months.

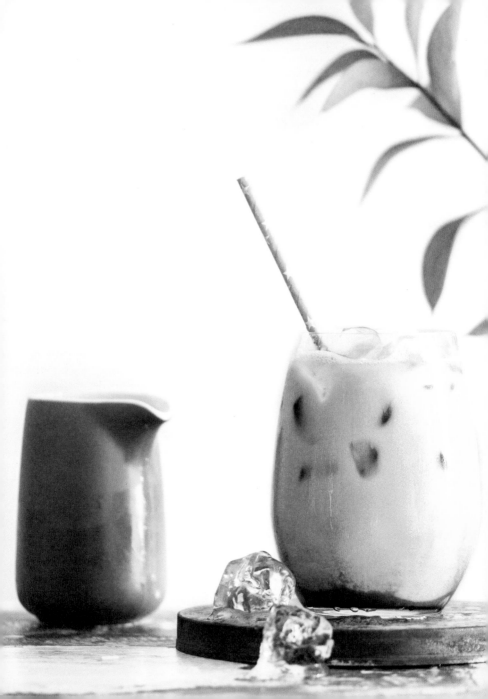

CBD LIBATIONS & EDIBLES

These recipes use CBD to address many of the conditions at the top of our ailment checklist, such as anxiety, difficulty sleeping, and mood disorders. You'll also find recipes for general supplementation. I have said it before and I'll say it again: CBD works differently with every body, so for internal ingestion, find your correct dose. Finding the dose that is right for you will ensure you have the best experience with CBD.

If you are concerned about—or interested in—THC in your recipes, make sure you do your research and double-check what you are buying. The products on the regulated adult-use and medical cannabis markets have an incredible diversity of CBD to THC ratios available for purchase, and CBD with THC is not the same as hemp-derived CBD (with less than 0.2 or 0.3 percent THC depending on the country). In fact, the effects can be quite different. A combination of THC and CBD in varying ratios will address different things. In some instances, and for some conditions, THC might be more efficacious. The same can be said of CBD.

CALM-MIND NERVINE TEA

Recipe by Kristi Blustein, yogi, herbalist, aromatherapist, and founder of KHUS + KHUS

YIELD: 1 SERVING

Nervine herbs are known as relaxants and have the ability to soothe nerves and alleviate irritation and stress. In this recipe, some of these herbs come together to create a nerve tonic that gently reduces stress and anxiety. Most of these ingredients are a little off the beaten path. You will have the easiest experience shopping online for these beauties.

INGREDIENTS

2 tablespoons dried gotu kola

1 tablespoon dried passionflower

1 tablespoon dried skullcap

½ tablespoon ground cardamom pods

1 dose full-spectrum CBD tincture

Honey, to taste

DIRECTIONS

• Combine the dried herbs and mix thoroughly. Boil 1 cup of water. Measure out 1 tablespoon of the herb mixture. Steep covered for a minimum of 30 minutes.

• Strain the tea and add the CBD tincture. Add honey to taste. Drink before bed to promote rest, or during situations of high anxiety. You can also drink this tea throughout the day, up to three cups daily.

• Store any leftover or premade tea in glass jars and place them in the refrigerator. In Ayurveda, we recommend taking liquids at room temperature, as cold liquids can have a negative effect on the body. If you want to drink tea that you stored in the fridge, let it sit at room temperature for 10–15 minutes before consuming. I know that this might seem a bit rigid, but don't stress and allow for some flexibility in the practice as it will result in a better outcome.

COMPLEMENTARY INGREDIENTS

Gotu kola is an herb used for anxiety, mental fatigue, and irritability. It's been known to promote nerve development. Passionflower is known for its sedative abilities and is ideal for insomnia, overstimulation of the mind, and stress-related headaches. Skullcap is ideal for calming you down from strong emotions such as anger and has a sattvic quality, meaning it offers equilibrium, clarity of perception, balance, and divine wisdom and ultimately promotes awareness and clarity. Cardamom is one of the best-known digestives in Ayurvedic medicine and can assist in the absorption of plant compounds into the body.

MATCHA SUNRISE

Recipe by Jessica Manley, a cannabis industry veteran, cofounder of Aplós, and founder of Healing Ventures

YIELD: 1 SERVING

Having worked with some of the biggest names in cannabis, Jessica is no stranger to a fast pace and the need to decompress and destress. This morning concoction utilizes Ayurvedic principles to create a potion with a symphony of beneficial effects greater than its individual parts. Drink for a calm, steady, yet alert start to your day.

INGREDIENTS

1 cup hemp, oat, or nut milk

2 teaspoons matcha

½ teaspoon ashwagandha powder

1 teaspoon coconut oil or ghee

1 teaspoon grass-fed butter

1 dose CBD tincture

1 teaspoon honey, coconut butter, or maple syrup

Dash of black or white pepper

Note: Ceremonial-grade matcha will amplify the effects of this drink and is recommended.

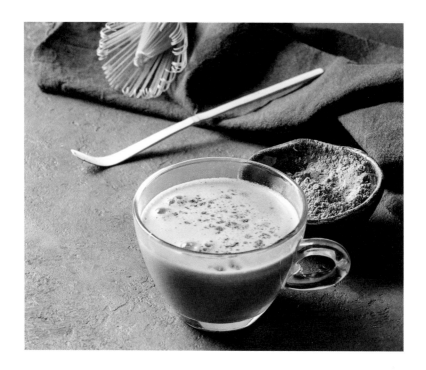

DIRECTIONS

• Warm the milk. Put all the ingredients into a blender and blend until thoroughly combined. Pour the beverage into your favorite vessel, and enjoy as a gentle spark moves into your system.

COMPLEMENTARY INGREDIENTS
Ashwagandha is one of Ayurveda's key botanicals and has similar effects as CBD: It boosts your mood and reduces stress and anxiety.

POTION OF THE GODS

Recipe by Danniel Swatosh is a cofounder and cannabis activist at Humble Bloom

YIELD: APPROXIMATELY 20 SERVINGS

This sweet and stimulating drink awakens the entire body with a delicate buzz that amplifies all the senses. High in anandamide, cacao has a mood-enhancing effect, softening the facial muscles and promoting a feeling of happiness or contentment.

INGREDIENTS

1 cup raw unsweetened cacao powder

8 teaspoons cinnamon

4 teaspoons Himalayan salt

4 teaspoons vanilla extract

20 doses CBD extract

For each serving:

1 cup (8 oz) plant-based milk or water

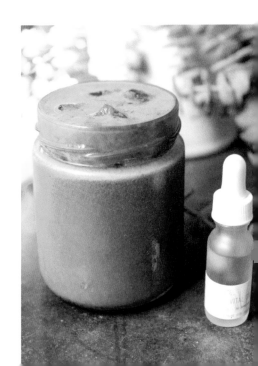

DIRECTIONS

• Mix all ingredients (except the milk or water) very well, making sure there are no clumps. Store in the fridge in a glass jar for up to 1 month.

• To make the drink, add 1 tablespoon of the mixture to your favorite plant-based milk or water. Shake or blend for a delicious drink that will take you to a place of such pleasure.

Note: The mixture (without the milk or water) can be used as a face mask. It will stimulate circulation, fight free radical damage, and reduce blemishes, helping to smooth fine lines and give you a rosy glow. Simply mix 1 tablespoon of the mixture with distilled water to make a paste; apply evenly to your face, letting it sit on the skin until dry.

COMPLEMENTARY INGREDIENTS

Cacao is the star complementary ingredient in this recipe. Danniel explains, "Cacao enters your body through your endocannabinoid receptors just like cannabis, opening your heart center with its main active compound, theobromine; dilating the blood vessels; and sending an array of 'feel good' chemicals to the brain. Cacao coupled with cannabis stimulates and awakens the entire body, creating a delicate buzz that amplifies all the senses."

ROSEMARY–LEMON SPRITZ

Recipe by Brandie Leach, founder of Sativa Science Club

YIELD: 4 SERVINGS

This is an excellent mocktail for a lazy summer evening with friends or a romantic summer night with your significant other. It is rich in terpenes and a pure delight for the senses. Sublingual cannabis consumption delivers active compounds directly to the bloodstream, so expect to experience the effects of your dosing quickly after consuming.

INGREDIENTS

1 cup honey

4 tablespoons dried rosemary

4 cups spring water, divided

4 doses water-soluble CBD extract or CBD tincture

1½ cups freshly squeezed lemon juice

½ tablespoon freshly grated lemon zest

A few lemon slices

Ice cubes

Soda water (optional)

Rosemary sprig, to garnish

Lemon twist, to garnish

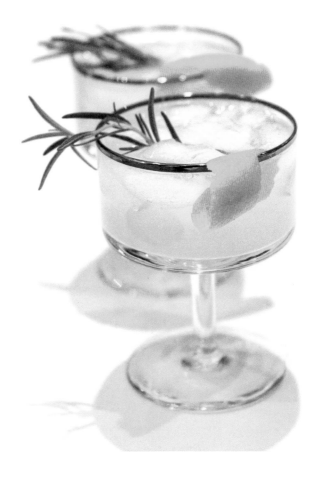

Note: You can substitute the rosemary with 4 tablespoons dried lavender flowers or pine needles, and use them as a garnish if you are looking for a more uplifting blend. To use an oil-based sublingual, simply add it as a garnish rather than during the shaking process. If you want to turn this recipe into a cocktail, add ⅔ of a shot (1 oz) of tequila or vodka, but please enjoy responsibly!

DIRECTIONS

• To make the syrup, mix your honey, rosemary, and 2 cups (16 oz) of spring water in a saucepan over medium heat. Bring the mixture to a rolling boil, then turn off the heat, let the mixture steep for about 10 minutes, and strain it with cheesecloth or a strainer fine enough to capture the rosemary. Place this mixture in the fridge until completely cool.

• When the syrup is ready, mix it with your lemon juice and add 2 more cups (16 oz) of spring water.

• For this next step, you'll need a martini shaker. If you don't have one, a mason jar with a lid will do. In your shaking apparatus, add lemon zest, lemon slices, an ice cube or two, and your tincture. Give your martini shaker a nice 30-second shake. Pour it over ice, add soda water to fill if desired, and garnish with a lemon twist and rosemary sprig.

COMPLEMENTARY INGREDIENTS

Lemons are chock-full of the terpene limonene. Limonene, also found in citrus rind oil, has long been used by naturalists for its anti-bacterial properties, but it is also known to elevate mood and uplift the mind. Even better, studies have shown that limonene may even increase the absorption of other terpenes. Rosemary contains the BCP (beta-caryophyllene) terpene. BCP is said to interact with receptors in the body, and specifically brain, potentially improving circulation and cognitive clarity. You can't go wrong combining this with the calming floral undertones of linalool, another beautiful balancing terpene found in lavender flower.

FLOWER MOON ELIXIR

Recipe by Erin Willis, holistic nutritionist and founder of Mother Indica

YIELD: 6 SERVINGS

This sparkling, zesty elixir makes a beautiful drink for a refreshing and relaxing vibe.

INGREDIENTS

3 bags sweet rose tea

2 bags hibiscus tea

1 bag white mulberry tea

6 cups ginger kombucha or soda water

6 doses CBD tincture

Fresh seasonal fruit for garnish

DIRECTIONS

• Place the tea bags in 3 cups of boiling water. (A mason jar is perfect for this.) You can steep the tea bags from 30 minutes to several hours.

• Squeeze the tea bags and discard them. Cool the tea with ice and store in the refrigerator. This is your base tea.

• For each serving, combine ½ cup of the iced base tea with 1 cup of kombucha or soda water and top with 1 dose of CBD tincture. Garnish with your favorite seasonal fruit.

MEZCAL MARGIE

Recipe by Elliott Coon and AdrinAdrina, the cofounders of Gem & Bolt Mezcal

YIELD: 1 SERVING

In this modern twist to the traditional margarita and fizz, the lovely women behind Gem & Bolt Mezcal have developed a fun cocktail with a powerful punch. This drink is also vegan and uses aquafaba, a foam created by whipping the starchy liquid from a can of chickpeas, as an alternative to whipped egg whites, which are common in traditional fizzes.

INGREDIENTS

Ice

2 ounces mezcal

1 ounce fresh lime juice

¾ ounce agave syrup

4 mint leaves plus additional leaves for garnish

¾ ounce aquafaba

1 dose CBD extract

Note: A CBD extract that is water soluble or alcohol-based will mix into the beverage. You can also use an oil-based extract; it will float on the top of the beverage, acting more like a garnish. If you use an oil-based product, make sure not to serve your beverage in plastic, as the oil will cling to the sides of the cup.

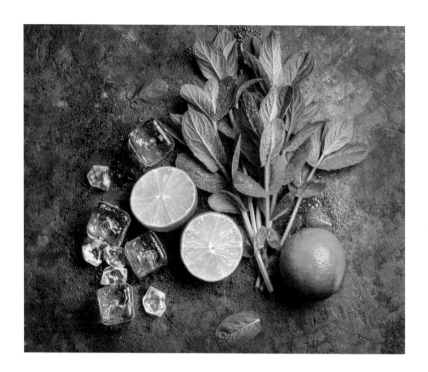

DIRECTIONS

• Fill a cocktail shaker or mason jar with a lid with ice. Add the mezcal, lime juice, agave, and 4 mint leaves. Shake vigorously. Strain into a coupe glass. Top with aquafaba and CBD oil. Garnish with a mint leaf.

COMPLEMENTARY INGREDIENTS
Mint contains myrcene, a terpene known for enhancing or modulating the effects and potency of other terpenes.

HEMP SEED TABBOULEH

Recipe by Megan Villa, Grace Saari, and Monica Campana, the founders of Svn Space

YIELD: 4 SERVINGS

This vegan, nut-free recipe is a high-protein hemp version of the well-loved Mediterranean and Middle Eastern salad tabbouleh. Enjoy it with fresh, warm pita bread, and for a little extra yumminess, you can add avocado.

INGREDIENTS

1 cup fresh parsley

½ cup fresh mint leaves

¼–½ teaspoon sea salt

3 large red vine tomatoes, chopped

1 cup hemp seed hearts

2 tablespoons hemp oil

2 tablespoons freshly squeezed lemon

Dash of lemon pepper

4 doses CBD oil

DIRECTIONS

• In a food processor, process parsley, mint, and sea salt until minced. (If you don't have a food processor, just chop everything really finely.) Transfer mixture to a large mixing bowl. Add the chopped tomatoes, hemp seeds, hemp oil, lemon juice, and lemon pepper.

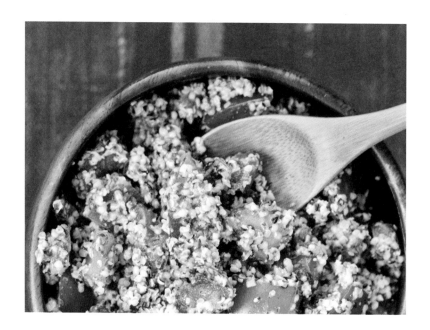

• Mix well. If you like, refrigerate for 30 minutes so the juices from the tomatoes can be absorbed. Before serving, add one dose of CBD oil to each portion.

COMPLEMENTARY INGREDIENTS

Lemons contain a concentration of limonene, a terpene known to relieve stress, elevate mood, and potentially increase the absorption of other terpenes. Hemp seeds and hemp oil not only are rich in omega-3 fatty acids and protein but also help give you the entourage effect (see page 24).

CITRUS CURRIED CHICKPEA & WILDFLOWER QUINOA SALAD

Recipe by Erin Willis, holistic nutritionist and founder of Mother Indica

YIELD: 4 SERVINGS

This fresh and lively salad packs a strong nutritional punch. Erin says, "This here salad is my go-to for whenever I feel overwhelmed with both depression and anxiety, when I can feel processed junk is running through my body, and when I want to feel my absolute best."

INGREDIENTS

2 cups dried chickpeas, soaked overnight in filtered water

1 cup quinoa, rinsed

2 cups vegetable broth

Sea salt, to taste

3 tablespoons olive oil

1 tablespoon turmeric powder

Freshly ground black pepper to taste

Smoked paprika, cumin, or other spices of your choice to taste (optional)

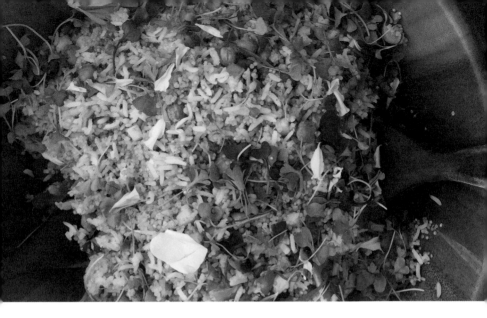

For the dressing:

2 tablespoons orange juice, freshly squeezed

1 tablespoon apple cider vinegar

1 tablespoon Dijon mustard

2 teaspoons raw honey

3 tablespoons olive oil

Turmeric, salt, and freshly ground pepper to taste

Spices such as paprika or cumin to taste (optional)

For assembly:

1 whole cucumber, diced

1 whole orange or yellow bell pepper, seeded and diced

1 whole red onion, diced

2–3 tablespoons edible flowers and/or microgreens

DIRECTIONS

• Drain and air dry the soaked chickpeas.

• Preheat oven to 350°F (120°C). While the oven is preheating, cook the rinsed quinoa in vegetable broth and sea salt until tender, about 25–30 minutes. Transfer to a large bowl, fluff with a fork, and let cool.

• While the quinoa is cooking, in a medium bowl mix the soaked chickpeas with the olive oil, turmeric, salt, and freshly ground black pepper. Bonus points for adding a dash of enticing spices like smoked paprika or cumin.

• On a cookie sheet lined with aluminum foil, spread the chickpeas evenly and bake for 35–40 minutes or until golden brown, giving the sheet a wiggle midway through for more of an even cook.

• While the chickpeas bake, prep the dressing by combining all ingredients except the olive oil. Once evenly mixed, slowly add in the olive oil; this will allow it to emulsify more easily. Once all the cooked goods are cooled, start assembling your salad to your liking by tossing the quinoa, chickpeas, dressings, and remaining ingredients together and enjoy!

COMPLEMENTARY INGREDIENTS
Citrus fruits contain limonene, which we have referenced earlier. When it is consumed often, it helps promote a healthy gut.

CBD GODDESS DRESSING

Recipe by Romany Pope, herbalist, Kundalini yoga teacher, and reiki practitioner

YIELD: 4 SERVINGS

This delicious dressing gives you an easy way to incorporate the healing properties of hemp into your everyday routine. It makes raw broccoli and beets taste like a treat! While it is called a dressing, you can also use it as a spread, a sauce, or a marinade. It can be used in any number of ways to enhance many kinds of foods—think grain bowl, sandwich, sautéed vegies, and more.

INGREDIENTS

3 tablespoons tahini

1 clove garlic

1 teaspoon miso

1 teaspoon raw local honey
or maple syrup

1 tablespoon cider vinegar

1 tablespoon water (or more if
needed)

Dash of cracked black pepper

4 doses CBD oil

DIRECTIONS

• Add all ingredients to a high-speed blender. Blend on high for 30 seconds or until smooth. If the blender is struggling, slowly add a small amount of water until the mixture flows better.

CBD ZUCCHINI MUFFINS

Recipe by Dr. Amanda Reiman, PhD, MSW, community director of Flow Kana, and member of the Cannabis Regulatory Commission in Oakland, California

YIELD: 12 SERVINGS

These healthy zucchini CBD muffins from Dr. Reiman can help combat post-workout muscle fatigue. A lifelong athlete, Dr. Reiman was diagnosed with osteoarthritis in her feet. She says, "Edibles are the best treatment for my arthritis, especially when preparing for a workout. They are long-lasting and positively impact the entire body. I like to have one muffin about an hour before my workouts."

INGREDIENTS

1⅔ cups whole-wheat pastry flour

1 cup brown sugar

1 teaspoon baking soda

½ teaspoon baking powder

¼ teaspoon cinnamon

¼ teaspoon salt

1 teaspoon vanilla

2 eggs

½ cup coconut oil, melted

12 servings CBD extract*

2 freshly grated zucchinis

⅔ cup dark chocolate chips

*Potency of the CBD extract is important here as adding too much liquid to this recipe will throw off the ratios of the other ingredients. It is best to use a high-potency oil to avoid adding extra liquid to the recipe. If you use a low-potency oil, you may need to adjust the amount of melted coconut oil.

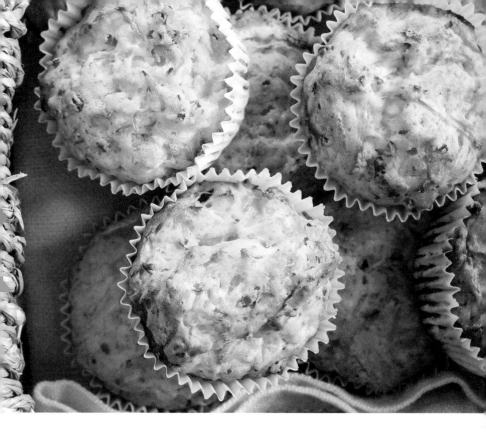

DIRECTIONS

• Preheat the oven to 350°F (175°C). In a large bowl, mix together the flour, sugar, baking soda, baking powder, cinnamon, and salt. Add the vanilla and eggs and mix the batter until fluffy. Add the coconut oil, CBD, and zucchini, and combine. Fold in the chocolate chips.

• Grease a muffin tin and add batter to each cup, filling each one until it is three-quarters full. Bake for 15–18 minutes, until the tops of the muffins are golden. Cool before removing the muffins from the tin.

STRAWBERRY SMOOTHIE FOR THE MICROBIOME

  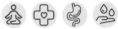

Recipe by Dr. Mollie Parker Szybala, naturopath and gut biome specialist at Sun Valley Natural Medicine

YIELD: 1 SERVING

The word *microbiome* refers to the trillions of microscopic organisms that live in our gut and work to optimize our digestion, metabolism, and immune health; regulate our mood; and do so much more. Our microbiomes need fiber to survive and are fueled by the fruit, greens, and seeds found in this recipe. The collagen in this smoothie is a powerful protein source that is said to relieve joint pain and prevent bone loss. It is also great for plumping the skin and helping its cellular structure.

INGREDIENTS

1 cup frozen strawberries

½ banana

1 cup organic kefir

1-inch knob fresh ginger, peeled

1 tablespoon chia seeds

2 tablespoons collagen hydrolysate powder

1 cup spinach

1 dose CBD extract

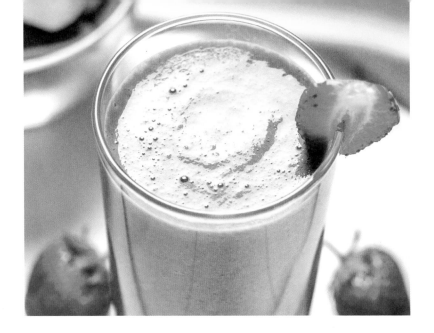

DIRECTIONS

• Place all the ingredients in a blender and add water until just covered. Blend until smooth.

COMPLEMENTARY INGREDIENTS

Kefir, which is rich in probiotics, or healthy bacteria, can help to replenish and restore our gut microbiome. The addition of ginger and CBD helps to reduce intestinal inflammation and promote healthy bowel movements. Collagen hydrolysate is a good source of protein that can help stabilize blood sugar, and, if you have leaky gut, heal the gut lining.

COCONUT CANDIES

   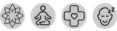

Recipe by Michelle Helfner, acupuncturist, Chinese medicine practitioner, and meditation expert

YIELD: 16 CHOCOLATES, SERVING SIZE OF 2–4 PER DAY

This healthy chocolate treat gives you a daily dose of CBD as well as a bit of relaxation and peacefulness. Michelle developed this recipe for her father, who was diagnosed with Alzheimer's disease. She explains, "I'm an advocate of food as medicine. In today's times, there are so many ways to get the nourishment that our bodies need without taking so many pills. My dad hated pills and loved chocolates, so I created a win-win solution. . . . It became the most pleasurable 'medicine' of the day."

INGREDIENTS

½ cup dried cranberries and/or raisins

Handful of mixed nuts (optional)

1 cup coconut oil

½ cup chia seeds (optional)

3 tablespoons fine cacao powder

3 tablespoons sweetener of your choice, such as honey, dates, stevia, or sugar

¼ teaspoon vanilla extract

16 doses of CBD extract

DIRECTIONS

• Line one ice cube tray with the dried fruit and nuts, if using.

• Mix the remaining ingredients in a blender and blend until creamy and smooth. Pour the mixture into the ice cube trays, filling up each cavity halfway with the mixture. Add your daily dose of CBD oil to each candy. Freeze for 30–60 minutes. Store in the fridge. These will last up to 2 weeks in the fridge and 3 months in the freezer.

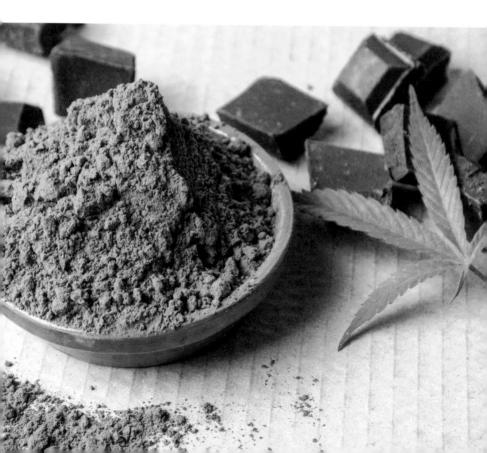

HAPPY TUMMY CBD GUMMIES

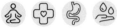

Recipe by Dr. Mollie Parker Szybala, naturopath and gut biome specialist at Sun Valley Natural Medicine

YIELD: 16 SERVINGS, 1 GUMMY PER SERVING

These tasty gummies are not your traditional treat—they are chock-full of reparative anti-inflammatories from ginger to turmeric and of course CBD. From a simple daily supplement to support overall daily function to a treatment for an upset stomach, this recipe is worth a try. We all need a little boost from time to time, and this is just the ticket.

INGREDIENTS

2½ cups water

2 tablespoons fresh turmeric, chopped

2 tablespoons fresh ginger, chopped

2 tablespoons lemon juice

2 tablespoons raw honey

16 doses CBD oil

1½ tablespoons organic gelatin powder

DIRECTIONS

• Add the water, turmeric, and ginger to a small pot. Bring the mixture to a boil and simmer for 15–20 minutes.

• Remove from the heat and stir in lemon juice, honey, and CBD. While it is still warm, add the water and then the gelatin powder, whisking immediately to prevent clumping.

• Pour the mixture into an 8 × 8-inch baking dish or a candy mold. If you use a mold, try to find one that allows for multiples of 16, so you know the volume of CBD per mold. Refrigerate for at least 30 minutes, until it is firm to the touch. If you used a baking dish, cut the slab into 16 equal squares. Cover tightly and consume within 3 days.

COMPLEMENTARY INGREDIENTS

The ginger and turmeric have not only synergistic effects that support each other but also strong anti-inflammatory properties. They aid proper digestion and support a healthy microbiome. Organic gelatin provides additional amino acids and the protein collagen, both of which promote fast healing of the GI tract.

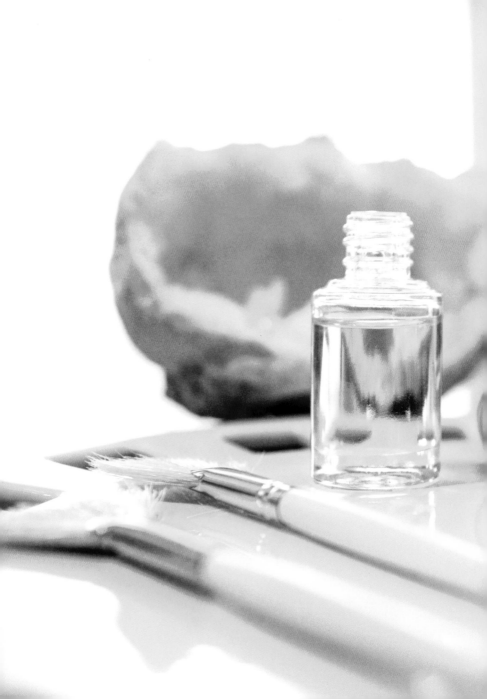

CBD BODY CARE

CBD formulations that are applied on your skin are a great way to address topical inflammation and achieve relief from acute and superficial conditions. Internationally distributed products largely focus on skincare, beauty, and pain relief, so I have collected a selection of recipes that speak directly to those areas of interest. The recipes contain complementary ingredients, such as carrier bases that have their own added benefits, essential oils that have terpenes that work synergistically with CBD, and so on. Remember, as with the other recipes, using more is not always better.

Unlike some products sold on shelves, these recipes do not use harsh chemical penetrators and synthetic preservatives. While that is beneficial for health purposes and makes these DIY recipes easy to make, please keep in mind that natural ingredients have a shelf life. Best-case scenario for recipes that have sat for a while, they will be less effective; worst case scenario, you could have an adverse reaction. Date all your finished products, and throw them out when their time is up!

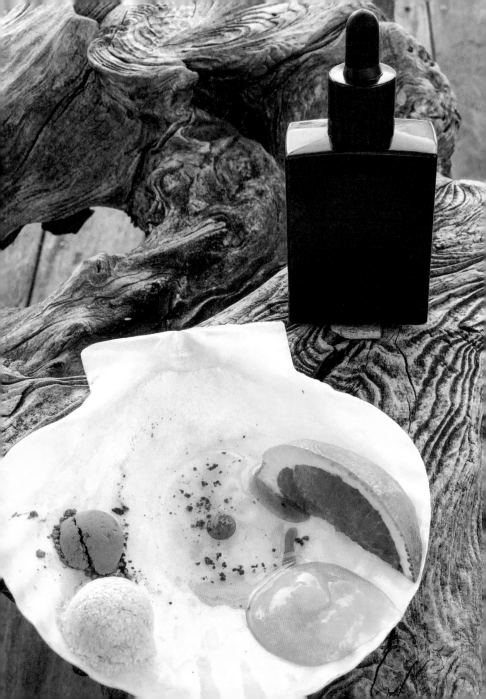

CBD BEAUTY FACE MASK

Recipe by Marysia Miernowska, herbalist, formulator, and cofounder of Rituel

YIELD: 1 APPLICATION

Made with superfoods, soothing oils, and replenishing rose flower water, this deeply nourishing and healing face mask has some of nature's finest anti-inflammatory ingredients and soothes skin irritations, redness, or puffiness. Unlike store-bought masks, which are filled with preservatives, this mask is nontoxic, edible, and rich in vitamins D, E, C, A, and B, leaving you with velvety smooth, clear, luminous, and radiant skin.

INGREDIENTS

½ teaspoon matcha

½ teaspoon rosewater

1 dose CBD oil

1 wedge organic orange, peeled

1 teaspoon organic raw honey

1 teaspoon vitamin E oil

DIRECTIONS

• Thoroughly wash and clean your face. Pat dry. Mix all the ingredients into a runny paste, and this massage lovingly onto your face using a circular motion and with an appreciation for the gifts from the healing plants and the luxurious ingredients in this mask. Relax for 20 minutes, rest, and receive. Rinse with water, and gently pat your face dry.

CREAMY HERBAL CBD MASSAGE OIL

Recipe by Yvonne Perez Emerson, founder of Make & Mary

YIELD: 12 APPLICATIONS

Combining calming plants in a massage oil takes the ritual of massage to the next level. This folk recipe for massage oil is a favorite of Yvonne.

INGREDIENTS

2 tablespoons dried chamomile

2 tablespoons dried comfrey

2 tablespoons dried lavender

2 tablespoons dried calendula

1 cup apricot or almond oil (add more to cover if needed, see directions)

For each cup of herbal oil:

¼ cup cocoa butter

½ cup coconut oil

6 doses sublingual CBD oil (in MCT base oil)

10–15 drops of essential oil of your choice (start with fewer and add more to desired saturation level)

DIRECTIONS

• Put all of the herbs in a wide-mouth glass jar. Use a wooden spoon to press the herbs down. Cover the herbs completely with the apricot or almond oil, adding more oil than the recipe calls for if recommended amount doesn't fully cover the herbs.

• Let the mixture sit in a warm place for 3–4 weeks. I like to put mine on a sunny windowsill. Alternatively, you can use a double boiler or slow cooker. If using a double boiler, place the herbs and oil in the jar and put the jar into a pot of warm water on the stove. Slowly heat the mixture to a low simmer. Do not overheat. Keep on low heat for about 2–3 hours. If using a slow cooker, place the mixture into the crock and keep it on low overnight, up to 8 hours.

• When the oil has infused, strain your herbs with a fine cheesecloth. For a cleaner oil, strain it several times.

• Mix the infused oil with the cocoa butter, coconut oil, and CBD oil. Warm these ingredients together on low heat until they are blended, then add your essential oil. Pour your creamy massage oil into wide-mouth mason jars or amber-colored jars. When stored in a cool, dark place, the oil should last for up to 6 months. Be careful to use clean hands when removing the oil from the jar for use. This will make it last longer by protecting it from contaminants.

Note: You can add a few more drops of essential oil after the mixture has cooled to at least 145°F (65°C). Lavender or ylang ylang are my favorite oils. Rose is also nice! Experiment with your own scents.

CBD HOT-OIL HAIR TREATMENT

Recipe by Raeven Duckett, cofounder of Community Gardens and board member of Supernova Women

YIELD: 1 APPLICATION

This treatment softens hair, and the CBD helps soothe scalp inflammation. Not only will it treat brittle hair, it will also stimulate blood flow in your scalp. Think of this as a spa treatment for your head, scalp, and hair. You will need a hot-oil applicator, which should be available readily online.

INGREDIENTS

1 dose CBD oil

½ tablespoon dried lavender

2 cups coconut oil

4 cups water

DIRECTIONS

• Combine all the ingredients in a slow cooker. Cook on low for 6–8 hours, stirring with a whisk hourly. Monitor the liquid level and add water as needed so there are always at least 3 cups (24 oz) of water in the pot.

• Pour the liquid into a large bowl, using cheesecloth to strain the lavender buds. Then pour a large kettle of boiling water, about 3–5 (24–40 oz) cups, over the cheesecloth and into a bowl to wash through any extra oil clinging to the plant material. Allow the plant material to cool, then squeeze out as much liquid as possible before discarding.

• Chill the mixture, allowing the fats to rise to the top. The oil will harden into a solid, making it easy to separate it from the water below. Rinse the solidified oil with cold water to wash away any leftover plant material. Place the solidified oil in the applicator.

• To apply, shampoo hair; hot-oil treatments are best absorbed on a clean scalp. Heat the hot-oil applicator in a cup of hot water. Let it sit in the water for 5 minutes, or until the oil has melted. Part the hair and apply the oil directly to your scalp. It's best to apply the oil, one section at time, starting from the back of your head and coming up to the front.

• Once you have applied the oil to your entire scalp, massage the oil into your scalp using your fingers for 3–5 minutes. Place a plastic shower cap on your hair for at least 30 minutes or, for a deeper experience, overnight. Rinse out with cold water.

COMPLEMENTARY INGREDIENTS
Both lavender and coconut oil promote healthy hair growth. Plus, lavender smells great and has relaxing effects.

HEMPSLEY'S CBD-INFUSED BEDTIME BALM

Recipe by Kristen Williams, founder of Hempsley and cannabis educator

YIELD: 6 OUNCES

This nourishing and relaxing balm supports sleep and deep relaxation. It can be used for massage or as a lip balm. Essential oils are optional, but grapefruit, peppermint, and ginger are great choices for lip balm. You can use 150 milligrams for mild relief or add up to 500 milligrams for more concentrated effects.

INGREDIENTS

½ cup unrefined coconut oil

¼ cup beeswax pellets

1 tablespoon hemp oil

Up to 500 milligrams CBD oil

1 teaspoon jojoba oil

Essential oils (optional)

DIRECTIONS

• Combine coconut oil and beeswax pellets in a double boiler and melt the mixture.

• Meanwhile, prepare containers to hold your balm and place them nearby. I like to use metal tins or glass. (Plastic containers tend to leach toxins when heated elements are added to them.)

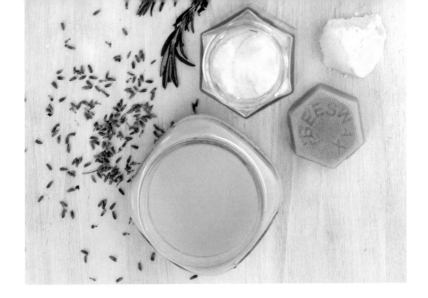

• Once the beeswax mixture has melted, add the hemp oil, CBD oil, jojoba oil, and essential oils, if using. Stir until incorporated. Pour the mixture into your prepared containers. The mixture will harden quickly, so make sure your containers are ready to go!

• Every night before bed, moisturize with this balm. The soles of your feet are a great place to start. Self-massage can help boost your endocannabinoid levels, relaxing you and signaling to your body that it's time for bed so that you can get truly deep, restful sleep. I find that when I do this, I fall asleep more quickly, sleep more deeply, and wake up feeling refreshed.

• When stored in a cool, dark place, the balm should last for up to 6 months. Be careful to use clean hands when removing the balm from the container for use. This will make it last longer by protecting it from contaminants.

EVAN'S SMOKE BLEND

Recipe by Evan Marshall, founder and CTO of Plain Jane

YIELD: 1 SERVING

CBD vape pens are quite widely available alongside tinctures, oils, and such. Vapes serve a function, as we mentioned earlier on page 56, in delivering medicine immediately for the most rapid onset of effects. For some, they are the best option. That being said, they do not have the best reputation. Many vape pens have questionable carrier oils, and their delivery mechanisms can be manufactured using questionable materials such as plastic and metal. This recipe is a great alternate to vaping premade cartridges, and I like to think that the ritual of smoking is best honored in the process of grinding and rolling the flower directly.

INGREDIENTS

1 tablespoon CBD hemp flower

¼ teaspoon mullein

¼ teaspoon raspberry leaf

¼ teaspoon lotus leaf

Rolling papers

Note: I recommend a hemp-focused blend with 80–85 percent hemp and 15–20 percent other ingredients, such as in the ratio above. The quantity of other ingredients, such as raspberry and lotus leaf, will add to the blend's flavor profile while keeping the focus on CBD. The additives generally also burn very quickly, and this combined with the oil from the hemp gives the blend a more consistent burn.

DIRECTIONS

• Grind all ingredients and mix together thoroughly for the best experience. This blend can be smoked with rolling papers or through a smoking apparatus (preferably glass) for the most immediate and impactful results. It can also be vaporized using a vaporizer.

COMPLEMENTARY INGREDIENTS

Lotus leaf can have antidepressant effects. When combined with CBD, it can help you feel relaxed and calm while retaining a clear mind.

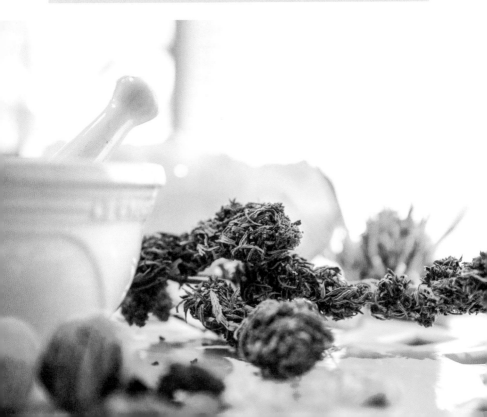

CONCLUSION

"I love cannabis because it is so intrinsically intertwined with us, creating homeostasis in our body so that all of its systems work in concert with one and the other. . . . It's the ultimate plant with the ability to give us just what we need. There is no other plant that can clothe, nourish, shelter, and enlighten us, plus heal our bodies, communities, and the planet."

–Danniel Swatosh, cofounder of Humble Bloom

People across cultures and traditions have been using cannabis, doing what works for them, and modifying those practices throughout history. Here we are now at the beginning of a post-prohibition era for cannabis, and we have the opportunity to recall, recover, reawaken, and honor past traditions and apply them to the present day.

All of the stories in this book about the use, success, or connection to cannabis—its medicinal applications and history—come from a place of compassion and knowledge. They represent opportunities to enact the principles and beliefs that are important in the process of reintegrating this momentarily forbidden plant back into our culture.

We can learn from the experiences of those who have used CBD— take note of the different trial periods and the varied experiences with conventional treatments that led many contributors in this book to find their own solutions with the cannabis plant. You may have a similar experience. Working with CBD is not a perfect science, but I want to encourage you to sample different recipes and brands and try different doses to address different ailments. When you can do this, when you can embrace this process, you will reach your own personal best, bringing a whole different kind of wellness into your life by incorporating intention, ritual, and ceremony. You will bring a fullness to your experience in ways you might never have anticipated.

The reverence with which we approach cannabis also leads us to important discussions. With the passage of recent laws, we now have not only a right to use CBD and, in some places, the entire cannabis plant itself, but also a duty to honor some of the important aspects of cannabis consumption. We can begin to reconstruct our view of cannabis to make it more inclusive and accessible for all, cultivating a relationship with the plant that allows us to grow it sustainably and providing fair and equal wages to the people working with the plant. Though these topics are heavy, you can't truly listen, be informed, or engage with the world if you don't "live in the process." This means you must remember to be fully present and engage with every piece of the conversation around cannabis, keeping your eyes, ears, and heart wide open.

Cannabis heals in so many ways. With its reemergence in the public eye, there are many opportunities to respect the plant's capabilities, remedy the injustices of the prohibition era, and heal our bodies. Having access to CBD is a part of a much bigger picture. It is an important part of a larger process, and it is a beautiful thing. Thank you for giving me the opportunity to tell a story about cannabis. Let's honor people's experience with cannabis in the past by taking it into the future with reverence.

Be well,
Blair

REFERENCES

Adams, Cydney. "The Man behind the Marijuana Ban for All the Wrong Reasons." CBS News, accessed November 16, 2019. https://www.cbsnews.com/news/harry-anslinger-the-man-behind-the-marijuana-ban/.

Ahmad, Hariri, Adam Gorka, Luke Hyde, Mark Kimak, Indrani Halder, Francesca Ducci, Robert Ferrell, David Goldman, and Stephen Manuck. "Divergent Effects of Genetic Variation in Endocannabinoid Signaling on Human Threat—and Reward—Related Brain Function." *Biological Psychiatry* 66, no. 1 (2009): 9–16. doi:10.1016/j.biopsych.2008.10.047.

Alger, Bradley E. "Getting High on the Endocannabinoid System." *Cerebrum: The Dana Forum on Brain Science*, November 1, 2013. https://www.ncbi.nlm.nih.gov/pmc/articles/PMC3997295/.

Andre, Christelle M., Jean-Francois Hausman, and Gea Guerriero. "*Cannabis Sativa*: The Plant of the Thousand and One Molecules." *Frontiers in Plant Science* 7, no. 19 (February 2016). https://www.ncbi.nlm.nih.gov/pmc/articles/PMC4740396/.

Anxiety and Depression Association of America. "Facts & Statistics." https://adaa.org/about-adaa/press-room/facts-statistics.

Basavarajappa, Balapal. "Critical Enzymes Involved in Endocannabinoid Metabolism." *Protein & Peptide Letters* 14, no. 3 (2007): 237–246. doi:10.2174/092986607780090829.

Baum, Dan. *Smoke and Mirrors: The War on Drugs and the Politics of Failure.* New York: Little, Brown and Company, 1997.

Ben-Shabat, Shimon, Ester Fride, Tzviel Sheskin, Tsippy Tamiri, Man-Hee Rhee, Zvi Vogel, Tiziana Bisogno, Luciano De Petrocellis, Vincenzo Di Marzo, and Raphael Mechoulam. "An Entourage Effect: Inactive Endogenous Fatty Acid Glycerol Esters Enhance 2-arachidonoyl-glycerol Cannabinoid Activity." *European Journal of Pharmacology* 353, no. 1 (1998): 23–31. doi:10.1016/s0014-2999(98)00392-6.

Black, Lester. "How a Bunch of San Francisco Queers Got Us Medical Marijuana." *The Stranger*, June 19, 2019. https://www.thestranger.com/weed/2019/06/19/40516811/how-a-bunch-of-san-francisco-queers-got-us-medical-marijuana.

Brodwin, Erin. "The Truth about 'Microdosing,' Which Involves Taking Tiny Amounts of Psychedelics like LSD." *Business Insider*, January 30, 2017. https://www.businessinsider.com/microdosing-lsd-effects-risks-2017-1.

Campos, Marcelo. "Leaky Gut: What Is It, and What Does It Mean for You?" *Harvard Health Blog*, September 22, 2017, last modified October 22, 2019. https://www.health.harvard.edu/blog/leaky-gut-what-is-it-and-what-does-it-mean-for-you-2017092212451.

Centers for Disease Control and Prevention. "Sleep and Sleep Disorders: About Our Program." June 5, 2017. www.cdc.gov/sleep/about_us.html.

"Controlled Substance Law." HG.org. https://www.hg.org/control.html.

Convention for Limiting the Manufacture and Regulating the Distribution of Narcotic Drugs, entry into force July 9, 1933. *League of Nations Treaty Series*, vol. 139: 303. https://treaties.un.org/Pages/ViewDetails.aspx?src=TREATY&mtdsg_no=VI-8-a&chapter=6&clang=_en.

Crudele, John. "Feds Patented Medical Pot . . . While Fighting It." *New York Post*, September 11, 2013. https://nypost.com/2013/09/11/feds-patented-medical-marijuana-even-when-they-were-fighting-it/.

Dahlhamer, James, et al. "Prevalence of Chronic Pain and High-Impact Chronic Pain Among Adults - United States, 2016." *Morbidity and Mortality Weekly Report* 67, no. 36 (September 14, 2018):1001–1006. https://www.cdc.gov/mmwr/volumes/67/wr/mm6736a2.htm.

Dalal, Pronob K., and Manu Agarwal. "Postmenopausal Syndrome." *Indian Journal of Psychiatry* 57, no. 6 (2015): 222. doi:10.4103/0019-5545.161483.

De Laurentiis, Andrea, Hugo A. Araujo, and Valeria Rettori. "Role of the Endocannabinoid System in the Neuro-endocrine Responses to Inflammation." *Current Pharmaceutical Design* 20, no. 29 (2014): 4697–4706. https://www.ncbi.nlm.nih.gov/pubmed/24588819.

Desjardins, Jeff. "The 6,000-Year History of Medical Cannabis." *Visual Capitalist*, June 20, 2018. https://www.visualcapitalist.com/history-medical-cannabis-shown-one-giant-map/.

Desy, Margherita M., and Phaedra Scott. "Ropemakers for the Navy: Part II." USS Constitution Museum website, October 21, 2016. https://ussconstitutionmuseum.org/2016/10/21/ropemakers-navy-part-ii.

Dincheva, Iva, et al. "FAAH Genetic Variation Enhances Fronto-Amygdala Function in Mouse and Human." *Nature Communications* 6, no. 1 (2015). doi:10.1038/ncomms7395.

Drug Enforcement Administration Museum & Visitors Center. "Harry Jacob Anslinger." https://deamuseum.org/anslinger/in-charge/.

Drug Policy Alliance. "A Brief History of the Drug War." http://www.drugpolicy.org/issues/brief-history-drug-war.

——— "Debunking the 'Gateway' Myth." February 2017. https://www.drugpolicy.org/sites/default/files/DebunkingGatewayMyth_NY_0.pdf.

Fetters, K. Aleisha. "Can CBD Oil Improve Your Fitness Results?" *U.S. News & World Report*, May 11, 2018. https://health.usnews.com/wellness/fitness/articles/2018-05-11/can-cbd-products-improve-your-fitness-results.

Fine, Perry G., and Mark J. Rosenfeld. "The Endocannabinoid System, Cannabinoids, and Pain." *Rambam Maimonides Medical Journal* 4, no. 4 (October 2013): e0022. https://www.ncbi.nlm.nih.gov/pmc/articles/PMC3820295/.

Frawley, David, and Vasant Lad. *The Yoga of Herbs: An Ayurvedic Guide to Herbal Medicine*. Lotus Press: Twin Lakes, WI, 1986.

French, Laurence, and Magdaleno Manzanárez. *NAFTA & Neocolonialism: Comparative Criminal, Human & Social Justice*. University Press of America: Lanham, MD, 2004.

Frontline. "Marijuana Timeline." Public Broadcasting Service website, accessed January 6, 2020. https://www.pbs.org/wgbh/pages/frontline/shows/dope/etc/cron.html.

Gregorio, Danilo De, Ryan J. Mclaughlin, Luca Posa, Rafael Ochoa-Sanchez, Justine Enns, Martha Lopez-Canul, Matthew Aboud, Sabatino Maione, Stefano Comai, and Gabriella Gobbi. "Cannabidiol Modulates Serotonergic Transmission and Reverses Both Allodynia and Anxiety-like Behavior in a Model of Neuropathic Pain." *Pain* 160, no. 1 (2019) 136–150. doi:10.1097/j.pain.0000000000001386.

Group, Edward. "What Are Polyphenols?" Global Healing Center, June 30, 2014. https://www.globalhealingcenter.com/natural-health/what-are-polyphenols/.

Hall-Flavin, Daniel K. "Clinical Depression: What Does That Mean?" Mayo Clinic. May 13, 2017. https://www.mayoclinic.org/diseases-conditions/depression/expert-answers/clinical-depression/faq-20057770.

Havelka, Jacqueline. "Does CBD Help or Hinder Sleep?" Leafly website, June 13, 2019. https://www.leafly.com/news/strains-products/how-to-use-cbd-marijuana-for-sleep.

History.com editors. "War on Drugs." History website, updated December 17, 2019. https://www.history.com/topics/crime/the-war-on-drugs.

Hume, Carothers Wallace. Synthetic fiber. US Patent 2130948A, filed July 20, 1936. https://patents.google.com/patent/US2130948A/en.

Hurt, Lukas. "Meet Lumir Hanus, Who Discovered the First Endocannabinoid." Leafly website, December 14, 2016. https://www.leafly.com/news/science-tech/lumir-hanus-discovered-first-endocannabinoid-anandamide.

Jikomes, Nick, and Michael Zoorob. "The Cannabinoid Content of Legal Cannabis in Washington State Varies Systematically Across Testing Facilities and Popular Consumer Products." *Scientific Reports* 8, no. 1 (2018). doi:10.1038/s41598-018-22755-2.

Kiley, Brendan. "From 'Evil Mexican Plants' to Legalization—A Brief History of Local Reporting on Cannabis." *The Stranger*, September 25, 2015. https://www.thestranger.com/blogs/slog/2015/09/25/22904884/from-evil-mexican-plants-to-legalizationa-brief-history-of-local-reporting-on-cannabis.

Kumari, Sangita, Sachin Pundhir, Piyush Priya, Ganga Jeena, Ankita Punetha, Konika Chawla, Zohra Firdos Jafaree, Subhasish Mondal, and Gitanjali Yadav. "EssOilDB: A Database of Essential Oils Reflecting Terpene Composition and Variability in the Plant Kingdom." *Database* (2014). https://www.ncbi.nlm.nih.gov/pmc/articles/PMC4273207/.

Lallanilla, Marc. "Ayurveda: Facts About Ayurvedic Medicine." *LiveScience*, January 7, 2015. https://www.livescience.com/42153-ayurveda.html.

Lee, Martin A. *Smoke Signals: A Social History of Marijuana—Medical, Recreational, and Scientific*. Scribner: New York, 2012.

Lima, Naiana G., et al. "Anxiolytic-like Activity and GC-MS Analysis of (R)-(+)-Limonene Fragrance, a Natural Compound Found in Foods and Plants." *Pharmacology Biochemistry and Behavior* 103, no. 3 (2013): 450–454. doi:10.1016/j.pbb.2012.09.005.

Lu, Hui-Chen, and Ken Mackie. "An Introduction to the Endogenous Cannabinoid System." *Biological Psychiatry* 79, no. 7 (October 2015): 516–525. doi:10.1016/j.biopsych.2015.07.028.

Lynn, Becky K., Julia D. López, Collin Miller, Judy Thompson, and E. Cristian Campian. "The Relationship between Marijuana Use Prior to Sex and Sexual Function in Women." *Sexual Medicine* 7, no. 2 (2019): 192–197. doi:10.1016/j.esxm.2019.01.003.

Marcus, Jacqueline B. "Vitamin and Mineral Basics: The ABCs of Healthy Foods and Beverages, Including Phytonutrients and Functional Foods." *Culinary Nutrition*, 279–331. Academic Press: New York, 2013. doi:10.1016/b978-0-12-391882-6.00007-8.

Marzo, Vincenzo Di, and Fabiana Piscitelli. "The Endocannabinoid System and Its Modulation by Phytocannabinoids." *Neurotherapeutics* 12, no. 4 (2015): 692–698. doi:10.1007/s13311-015-0374-6.

Mayo Clinic staff. "How Stress Affects Your Body and Behavior." Mayo Clinic website, April 4, 2019. https://www.mayoclinic.org/healthy-lifestyle/stress-management/in-depth/stress-symptoms/art-20050987.

———. "Insomnia." Mayo Clinic website, accessed January 6, 2020. https://www.mayoclinic.org/diseases-conditions/insomnia/symptoms-causes/syc-20355167.

McPartland, John M., Isabel Matias, Vincenzo Di Marzo, and Michelle Glass. "Evolutionary Origins of the Endocannabinoid System." *Gene* 370, no. 29 (January 23, 2006): 64–71. https://www.sciencedirect.com/science/article/abs/pii/S0378111905007067?via=ihub.

"Medical Cannabis: A Short Graphical History: China." Antique Cannabis Book website accessed December 16, 2019. http://antiquecannabisbook.com/chap2B/China/China.htm.

Moore, Melissa. "How the Endocannabinoid System Was Discovered: Cannabis Sciences." LabRoots website, accessed April 05, 2018. https://www.labroots.com/trending/cannabis-sciences/8456/=endocannabinoid-system-discovered.

Nagarkatti, Prakash, Rupal Pandey, Sadiye Amcaoglu Rieder, Venkatesh L. Hegde, and Mitzi Nagarkatti. "Cannabinoids as Novel Anti-inflammatory Drugs." *Future Medicinal Chemistry* 1, no. 7 (2009): 1333–1349. doi:10.4155/fmc.09.93.

National Cancer Institute. "Diethylstilbestrol (DES) and Cancer." October 5, 2011. https://www.cancer.gov/about-cancer/causes-prevention/risk/hormones/des-fact-sheet

Newton, David E. *Marijuana: A Reference Handbook, 2nd Edition.* ABC-CLIO: Santa Barbara, CA, 2017.

Nunley, Kim. "Why Is Marijuana Illegal? A Look at the History of MJ in America." *Medical Marijuana, Inc. News*, July 28, 2019. https://www.medicalmarijuanainc.com/news/the-road-to-prohibition-why-did-america-make-marijuana-illegal-in-the-first-place/.

"The People's History." *The Thistle* 13, no. 2 (September/October 2000). https://www.mit.edu/~thistle/v13/2/history.html.

Peschel, Wieland. "Quality Control of Traditional Cannabis Tinctures: Pattern, Markers, and Stability." *Scientia Pharmaceutica* 84, no. 3 (April 18, 2016): 567–584. https://www.ncbi.nlm.nih.gov/pmc/articles/PMC5064247/.

Reefer Madness. Directed by Louis J. Gasnier. 1936. Motion Picture Ventures, 1938.

Robbins, Curt. "Understanding Terpenes: Myrcene." Strainprint Community website, February 22, 2019. https://strainprint.ca/community/cannabis-terpenes-myrcene/.

Ross, Michele. "Can Cannabis Replace ERT for Menopause?" LinkedIn, October 3, 2015. https://www.linkedin.com/pulse/can-cannabis-replace-ert-menopause-michele-noonan-ross-phd.

Ruhaak, Lucia Renee, Jenny Felth, Pernilla Christina Karlsson, Joseph James Rafter, Robert Verpoorte, and Lars Bohlin. "Evaluation of the Cyclooxygenase Inhibiting Effects of Six Major Cannabinoids Isolated from Cannabis Sativa." *Biological & Pharmaceutical Bulletin* 34, no. 5 (2011): 774–778. doi:10.1248/bpb.34.774.

Russo, Ethan B. ""CBD, the Entourage Effect & the Microbiome: Interview with Dr. Ethan Russo." By Marin A. Lee. Project CBD. January 7, 2019. https://www.projectcbd.org/science/dr-ethan-russo-cbd-entourage-effect-and-microbiome.

———. "Clinical Endocannabinoid Deficiency Reconsidered: Current Research Supports the Theory in Migraine, Fibromyalgia, Irritable Bowel, and Other Treatment-Resistant Syndromes." *Cannabis and Cannabinoid Research* 1, no. 1 (July 1, 2016): 154–165. doi:10.1089/can.2016.0009.

Sales, Amanda J., Carlos C. Crestani, Francisco S. Guimarães, and Sâmia R.L. Joca. "Antidepressant-like Effect Induced by Cannabidiol Is Dependent on Brain Serotonin Levels." *Progress in Neuro-Psychopharmacology and Biological Psychiatry* 86 (2018): 255–261. doi:10.1016/j.pnpbp.2018.06.002.

Schiff, I. *"Effects of Estrogens on Sleep and Psychological State of Hypogonadal Women."* JAMA 242, no. 22 (November 30, 1979): 2405–2407. doi:10.1001/jama.242.22.2405.

Schlosser, Eric. "Reefer Madness." *The Atlantic*, August 1994. https://www.theatlantic.com/magazine/archive/1994/08/reefer-madness/303476/.

———. *Reefer Madness: Sex, Drugs, and Cheap Labor in the American Black Market.* Houghton Mifflin: New York, 2003.

Shannon, Scott, Nicole Lewis, Heather Les, and Shannon Hughes. "Cannabidiol in Anxiety and Sleep: A Large Case Series." *The Permanente Journal* 23 (January 7, 2019): 18–41. doi:10.7812/tpp/18-041.

Single Convention on Narcotic Drugs, open for signature March 30, 1961. *United Nations Treaty Series*, vol. 520: 151. https://treaties.un.org/pages/ViewDetails.aspx?src=TREATY&mtdsg_no=VI-15&chapter=6.

Smith, Noah. "Cannabis Research Pioneer Hopes Latest Discovery Is Not Overlooked—Again." NBC News website, September 26, 2019. https://www.nbcnews.com/tech/innovation/cannabis-research-pioneer-hopes-latest-discovery-not-overlooked-again-n1059116.

"State Marijuana Laws in 2019 Map." Governing website. https://www.governing.com/gov-data/safety-justice/state-marijuana-laws-map-medical-recreational.html.

"Stress Symptoms: Physical Effects of Stress on the Body." WebMD, reviewed by Jennifer Casarella, August 1, 2019. https://www.webmd.com/balance/stress-management/stress-symptoms-effects_of-stress-on-the-body#1.

Sullum, Jacob. "'Mexican, Crazed by Marihuana, Runs Amuck with Butcher Knife.'" Reason.com, August 4, 2014. https://reason.com/2014/08/04/mexican-crazed-by-marihuana-runs-amuck-w/.

Szalay, Jessie. "What Are Flavonoids?" LiveScience website, October 20, 2015. https://www.livescience.com/52524-flavonoids.html.

Thompson, Matt. "The Mysterious History of 'Marijuana.'" NPR, July 22, 2013. https://www.npr.org/sections/codeswitch/2013/07/14/201981025/the-mysterious-history-of-marijuana.

Tilray. "Myrcene, Linalool, and Bisabolol: What Are the Benefits of These Cannabis Terpenes?" Leafly website, May 10, 2016. https://www.leafly.com/news/cannabis-101/myrcene-linalool-and-bisabolol-what-are-the-benefits-of-these-can.

U.S. Food and Drug Administration. "FDA Approves First Drug Comprised of an Active Ingredient Derived from Marijuana to Treat Rare, Severe Forms of Epilepsy." News release, June 25, 2018. https://www.fda.gov/news-events/press-announcements/fda-approves-first-drug-comprised-active-ingredient-derived-marijuana-treat-rare-severe-forms.

Vardanyan, R.S., and V.J. Hrudy. *Synthesis of Essential Drugs.* Elsevier Science: Amsterdam, 2006. https://www.sciencedirect.com/topics/chemistry/fluoxetine.

Vigil, Jacob, Sarah Stith, Jegason Diviant, Franco Brockelman, Keenan Keeling, and Branden Hall. "Effectiveness of Raw, Natural Medical Cannabis Flower for Treating Insomnia under Naturalistic Conditions." *Medicines* 5, no. 3 (July 11, 2018): 75. doi:10.3390/medicines5030075.

Wilcox, Anna. "The Origin of the Word 'Marijuana.'" Leafly website, August 14, 2019. https://www.leafly.com/news/cannabis-101/where-did-the-word-marijuana-come-from-anyway-01fb.

Williams, Adela, Jeremy Willcocks, Evelina Norwinski, Raqiyyah Pippins, and Silvia Valverde. "Update on the EU Regulation of CBD in Foods and Vaping." *BioSlice Blog*, July 3, 2019. https://www.biosliceblog.com/2019/07/update-on-the-eu-regulation-of-cbd-in-foods-and-cosmetics/.

Xiong, Wei, Tanxing Cui, Kejun Cheng, Fei Yang, Shao-Rui Chen, Dan Willenbring, Yun Guan, Hui-Lin Pan, Ke Ren, Yan Xu, and Li Zhang. "Cannabinoids Suppress Inflammatory and Neuropathic Pain by Targeting 3 Glycine Receptors." *Journal of Experimental Medicine* 209, no. 6 (2012): 1121–1134. doi:10.1084/jem.20120242.

Young, Saundra. "Marijuana Stops Child's Severe Seizures." CNN website, August 7, 2013. https://www.cnn.com/2013/08/07/health/charlotte-child-medical-marijuana/index.html.

Zou, Shenglong, and Ujendra Kumar. "Cannabinoid Receptors and the Endocannabinoid System: Signaling and Function in the Central Nervous System." *International Journal of Molecular Sciences* 19, no. 3 (2018): 833. doi:10.3390/ijms19030833.

ACKNOWLEDGMENTS

To the nameless and faceless warriors, to the advocates, to those just trying to get by, to those who were and are behind bars holding down the fort for us and making it possible for us to move forward through open windows of cannabis reform with cause and passion, I thank you. To those who use their status and their money to further the movement toward decriminalization and destigmatization of cannabis, I appreciate it. To those that have been villainized and disenchanted, there is hope. We are on a path that started many years before me and will continue on heartily with compassion much beyond me. There is hope that we can learn how to do this a better way. Until then, the efforts and the continuous fortitude in which you move forward with this movement are beyond expressible gratitude.

There is a South African word, *ubuntu*, which—much like the word *reverence*—is about honoring what came before you and knowing that you are where you are now because of all that was before you. It is an important part of what shapes the future. I cannot begin to thoroughly express my gratitude and motivation that have been made possible by those who came before me on this journey toward cannabis integration with all the words in the world or with as many actions as I can muster in a lifetime. I do intend to remain open to the responsibilities I am asking to take on and the opportunities that may present themselves and morph on this journey. I look forward to being able to further collaborate with all those who have made this possible, known and included in this book and not. Let this be an offering to keep the doors of collaboration and education open. Thank you all for doing what you do. Ubuntu.

INDEX

Forms and use methods (*continued*)

PICTURE CREDITS

© Yancy Caldwell: 43, 46, 74, 105, 122, 135

Getty Images: Belchonock 84, Creative-Family 121, Epine Art (orange) 60, Natasha Breen 101, Foxys Forest Manufacture 96, Nata Golubnycha 8, Наталия Гусарова (tree), IRA EVVA 18, Karandaev 109, Open Range Stock 54, Tashka2000 119, Pimpay (dropper) 60, Den Potisev (plant, flower) i 1, 60, Tainar viii, Xiefei x, Yellowdesign (juice) 60, Zzayko (powder, isolate) 60

© Kristin Williams Hempsley: 133

© Mother Indica, Erin Willis: 113

Shutterstock: Davooda 85 (calm icon throughout), HN Works (soothe icon throughout), iconohek (gut icon throughout), Katflare (wellness icon throughout), kuroksta (elevate icon throughout), Motorama (sleep & beauty icon throughout), Noch 75, Jordan Wende 51

Stockfood: © Asya Nurullina 85

Stocksy: Jeremy Pawlowski 50

© Photo by Rituel: 126

© Romany Pope: 102

© SVN Space: 4, 111

ABOUT THE AUTHOR

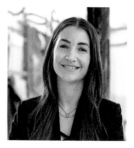

Blair Lauren Brown is the founder and CEO of Verté Essentials, a luxury wellness and beauty brand that has been featured in *Forbes* and *Cosmopolitan*, among other publications. Verté is one of the first brands to offer all-natural beauty and wellness products featuring cannabis hemp–derived CBD. She also founded the first luxury fine-jewelry company that is a certified B Corporation, and she makes it a point to integrate positive, sustainable environmental and humanitarian operations in every project she pursues, including both of these companies.

Blair's work with cannabis extends beyond the business and dates back to 2004, when she assisted medical grow operations that were founded in the wake of California's passage of Prop 215. Following a path of deep appreciation for the journey of cannabis culture through prohibition to present day, she advocates for a more progressive future. These efforts include her TEDx Sun Valley talk, called "Cannabis Mirror," where she explored the history of cannabis in the US as well as the study she developed and conducted on CBD and the naturally occurring cannabinoids in breast milk. She has also directed and produced *Burning Down the House: Queers and PWAs Lighting the Fire on Cannabis Legalization*, a documentary on the legalization of cannabis surrounding the AIDS/HIV epidemic.

As a certified advanced Sadhana yoga teacher, Blair has been able to combine her leadership in wellness practices with her cannabis experience and advocacy across the formulation, practice, and use of Verté products. She can be found teaching cannabis history, medicine, and ritual; Sadhana yoga; and other wellness practices at events and retreats across the US. Blair resides in New York City and Sun Valley, Idaho.